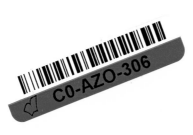

How to Find Information About AIDS

About the Authors

VIRGINIA A. LINGLE, MSLS, is Reference Librarian at the Milton S. Hershey Medical Center, College of Medicine, The Pennsylvania State University. She specializes in bibliographic instruction and the use of microcomputers in medical education. She is co-editor of the Medical Library Association publication entitled, *Public Services Section – MLA Newsletter*.

M. SANDRA WOOD, MLS, MBA, is Head, Reference, at the Milton S. Hershey Medical Center, College of Medicine, The Pennsylvania State University. She holds the academic rank of Librarian. In 1986, Ms. Wood was the recipient of the Ida and George Eliot Prize of the Medical Library Association for *Cost Analysis, Cost Recovery, Marketing, and Fee-Based Services*, the published work which has been judged most effective in furthering medical librarianship. She is the editor of *Medical Reference Services Quarterly*.

How to Find Information About AIDS

Virginia A. Lingle
M. Sandra Wood

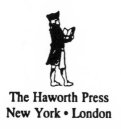

The Haworth Press
New York • London

The Haworth Press, Inc., 12 West 32 Street, New York, NY 10001
EUROSPAN/Haworth, 3 Henrietta Street, London WC2E 8LU England

Library of Congress Cataloging-in-Publication Data

Lingle, Virginia A.
    How to find information about AIDS.

    Bibliography: p.
    Includes indexes.
    1. AIDS (Disease) — Information services — Directories. 2. AIDS (Disease) —
Bibliography. I. Wood, M. Sandra. II. Title.
RC607.A26L56   1988   616.97'92'0072   88-758
ISBN 0-86656-752-6

CONTENTS

Introduction

The dissemination of information on acquired immune deficiency syndrome (AIDS) has become a major priority of the health care community in the last several years. The AIDS epidemic has grown beyond the scope of any single group in our society and has become a problem of national as well as worldwide proportions. For this reason, the attention of numerous groups and agencies has focused on this issue to produce a vastly increasing flow of information.

The purpose of this work is to assist the health professional and the general public alike in their efforts to tap into this information flow by providing an inexpensive resource to key access points such as government agencies, community hotlines, organizational resources, funding sources, major publications, and informational databases. This work can in no way be called comprehensive due to the large number of local organizations that exist and the new programs and services that are continually being developed.

National organizations are included in this listing if they provide some service to AIDS patients and their loved ones or if the organization distributes information about the AIDS crisis. An organization is excluded if it deals with issues relating only to homosexuality with no particular emphasis on AIDS. Local organizations are selectively included as a representation of the numerous community groups around the United States.

Health departments for each state and the District of Columbia are included as major access points within each respective state. Organizations that conduct research, as well as those that provide funding for research efforts, and government sources have been grouped into a single chapter because of the multiple roles of the federal government as a conductor of research, as a source for research funding, as a distributor of general information, and as a regulator of environmental issues, social security reimbursements, housing standards and more as they relate to AIDS. Hotlines were included as they could be identified. Computerized resources include online database, a computer database and a computer-assisted program, both for the IBM PC; bulletin boards; and a messaging system. Search of online databases for current developments in AIDS research is vital, so the emphasis of this chapter is on general biomedical and specialized AIDS databases. The selection of biomedical databases was made based on "hit" frequency in searching for AIDS information in BRS and DIALOG, two major database vendors.   Print sources of information represent a selection only of the materials available. An effort was made to cover most aspects of the disease, although the emphasis is on clinical information. The majority of the books listed have been published since 1985.   Popular literature was in most cases not considered for inclusion. Specialized journal titles include all that could be identified, although many more newsletters exist on the local level. Audiovisuals are listed by producer rather than by title only as a better means of identifying the resources available.

Virginia A. Lingle
M. Sandra Wood

    The authors gratefully acknowledge the help of Joan Bernardo, Robin Long, and the Reference Staff of the George T. Harrell Library; John Houck, M.D., Division of Otorhinolaryngology; and Peter S. Houts, Ph.D., Department of Behavioral Science, The M.S. Hershey Medical Center, The Pennsylvania State University, Hershey, PA.

Organizational Resources

Many organizations have been established or expanded in the past several years to deal with the AIDS epidemic. National organizations that have historically dealt with the issues of sexual health, homosexuality, blood products, and the chronically ill have refocused their services to include AIDS-related issues. Local groups are continually emerging to meet such needs as virus testing, counseling, education, and treatment. Several, more extensive directories exist for identifying local groups, for example, the U.S. Conference of Mayors *National Directory of AIDS-Related Services* and a directory of organizations published by the National AIDS Network. For this reason, the organizations listed here are more national in scope. However, a number of local organizations have been included as a representation of the types of groups that exist. Some of the national organizations have branch offices in each state, such as the American Red Cross, that can be utilized for information, as well.

Often, the groups identified with the term "project" in their names are local volunteer groups that provide a wide range of services. These include testing; counseling; the production and distribution of educational materials; publishing newsletters; providing support to AIDS/ARC patients, such as financial aid, clothing, housing, legal aid, social contacts, and transportation; maintaining referral lists of sympathic health care providers; conducting seminars and workshops; providing speakers; and staffing telephone hotlines. National organizations deal with many of the same aspects as well as performing functions of a broader scope such as lobbying Congress on AIDS-related issues, coordinating research efforts, and providing funding. Because many organizations provide a similar range of services, annotations have been provided only as a note of unique services or as a representation of the range of possible services.

Sources for identifying a local support group or information supplier include: (1) each of the state health departments, (2) the health departments of major cities around the U.S., (3) The National AIDS Network (see listing), or (4) the U.S. Conference of Mayors publication (see listing.) Updated information on national organizations appears annually in publications such as the *Encyclopedia of Associations* published by the Gale Research Company, or online in databases such as the DIRLINE file produced by the National Library of Medicine.

1

The terms "local" or "national" that appear in parentheses after the organization title indicate the geographic focus of the group. Most local groups will provide services for their respective states or will give referrals to another appropriate agency.

AID Atlanta (AIDA)   (Local)
811 Cypress Street
Atlanta, GA 30308
(404) 872-0600

AIDS   (Local)
Suite 700
1555 Wilson Boulevard
Rosslyn, VA 22209

> Distributes information to the general public such as the booklets, *The Surgeon General's Report; AIDS, Sex and You; AIDS and Children; and AIDS and Your Job: Are There Risks?*

AIDS Action Committee   (Local)
661 Boylston Street
Boston, MA 02116
(617) 437-6200

> Publishes the *AIDS Action Committee Update.*

AIDS Action Project   (Local)
Whitman-Walker Clinic
2335 18th Street NW
Washington, DC 20009
(202) 332-5295
(202) 332-AIDS

AIDS and KS Foundation/Sacramento   (Local)
2115 J Street
Suite 3
Sacramento, CA 95816
(916) 448-AIDS

AIDS Assistance Program   (Local)
P. O. Box 578418
Chicago, IL 60657
(312) 539-2437

AIDS CARE Project   (National)
University of South Carolina
School of Public Health
Columbia, SC 29208
(803) 777-2273

Research and education on AIDS.

AIDS Center of Queens County   (Local)
113-20 Jamaica Avenue
Richmond Hill, NY 11418
(718) 575-8855
(718) 847-1966

AIDS Education Project   (Local)
P. O. Box 4073
Key West, FL 33041
(305) 294-8302

Provides education and counseling.

AIDS Education Project of New Jersey Gay Coalition   (Local)
P. O. Box 1431
New Brunswick, NJ 08903
(201) 596-0767

AIDS Foundation of Chicago   (Local)
845 North Michigan Avenue
Suite 903E
Chicago, IL 60611
(312) 988-9005

AIDS Institute   (Local)
New York State Department of Health
Empire State Plaza
Corning Tower, Room 2580
Albany, NY 12237

AIDS Project   (Local)
48 Deering Street
Portland, ME 04101
(207) 774-6877

(207) 775-1267
(800) 851-AIDS

Maintains multiple services which include a speakers' bureau, hotline, educational materials, *The AIDS Project News*, counseling and testing, support groups, financial assistance, food and clothing banks.

AIDS Project/Los Angeles (Local)
7362 Santa Monica Boulevard
Los Angeles, CA 90046
(213) 876-8951
or
3670 Wilshire Boulevard
Suite 300
Los Angeles, CA 90010

Provides a program of support services for people with AIDS, their families and their loved ones through complete case management, housing, counseling, referrals, and more.

AIDS Project/Springfield (Local)
P. O. Box 8047
Springfield, MO 65801
(417) 864-8373

AIDS Reports (National)
P. O. Box 14252
Washington, DC 20044

Can write for free AIDS literature.

AIDS Resource Center, Inc. (National)
P. O. Box 792
Old Chelsea Station
New York, NY 10011
(212) 481-1270

Services include residential treatment and bereavement counseling.

AIDS Resource Foundation for Children (National)
385 C. Hulses Corner Road
Howell, NJ 07731

AIDS Resource Project of GROW   (National)
P. O. Box 4535
Wilmington, NC 28406

AIDS Response Program   (National)
12832 Garden Grove Boulevard
Suite E
Garden Grove, CA 92643
(714) 534-0961

AIDS Rochester, Inc.   (Local)
20 University Avenue
Rochester, NY 14605
(716) 232-3580
(716) 232-4430 (hotline)

> Provides advocacy services, food and clothing banks, crisis intervention, educational programs, emergency funds, 24-hour hotline, interpreters, newsletter *Awareness*, referrals, support groups, and transportation.

AIDS Task Force, Inc.   (Local)
P. O. Box 13527
Fort Wayne, IN 46869
(219) 483-8280

> Serves as an education and referral service.

Aliveness Project   (Local)
5307 Russell Street
Minneapolis, MN 55410
(612) 929-8256

American Association for Continuing Care   (National)
1101 Connecticut Avenue NW
Washington, DC 20036
(202) 857-1194

> Disseminates information about homecare.

American Association of Physicians for Human Rights   (National)
Box 14366
San Francisco, CA 94144
(415) 558-9353

Founded in San Francisco in 1981 for physicians and medical students for the elimination of discrimination in the health professions on the basis of sexual or affectional orientation, and for the delivery of supportive and unprejudiced medical care for gay and lesbian patients.

American Association of Sex Educators, Counselors, and Therapists
(National)
11 Dupont Circle NW
Suite 220
Washington, DC 20036
(202) 462-1171

Assists educational, religious, clinical, and social agencies in developing human relations and sex curricula; evaluates programs and advises on materials and human resources.

American Civil Liberties Union   (National)
Lesbian and Gay Rights Project
132 West 43rd Street
New York, NY 10036
(202) 944-9800

Offers a free publication, *AIDS: Basic Documents and Model Statutes.*

American College Health Association   (National)
Task Force on AIDS
15879 Crabbs Branch Way
Rockville, MD 20855
(301) 963-1100

American College of Obstetricians and Gynecologists   (National)
Resource Center
600 Maryland Avenue, SW, 300 East
Washington, DC 20024-2588
(202) 863-2518

Distributes information on women and AIDS.

American Federation of Home Health Agencies   (National)
1320 Fenwick Lane
Suite 500
Silver Spring, MD 20910
(301) 588-1454

Disseminates information on homecare.

American Foundation for the Prevention of Venereal Disease, Inc.
(National)
799 Broadway
Suite 638
New York, NY 10003
(212) 759-2069

Non-profit agency dependent on public support. Produces and disseminates information on sexually transmitted disease prevention.

American Health Consultants, Inc. (National)
67 Peach Park Drive, NE
Atlanta, GA 30309
(404) 351-4523

Publishes the *AIDS Alert.*

American Health Foundation (National)
320 East 43rd Street
New York, NY 10017
(212) 953-1900

American Hospital Association (National)
Resource Center
840 North Lake Shore Drive
Chicago, IL 60611
(312) 280-6263

Compiles bibliographies of selected current references on issues relevant to hospital administration. AIDS-related publications include a bibliography, *AIDS: Administrative Issues*, and the title *A Hospitalwide Approach to AIDS.*

American Life Lobby (ALL) (National)
P. O. Box 490
Stafford, VA 22554
(703) 659-4171

A nonprofit organization involved in research, publication, and dissemination of materials pertaining to a broad spectrum of medical issues including AIDS. Services are free, except for the cost of materials, and are available to anyone.

American Medical Association   (National)
Council on Scientific Affairs
Panel on Acquired Immunodeficiency Syndrome
535 N. Dearborn Street
Chicago, IL 60610
(312) 645-5000

American Medical Society on Alcoholism and Other Drug Dependencies
(National)
12 West 21st Street
New York, NY
(212) 206-6770

> Publishes free pamphlet: *Guidelines for Facilities: Treating Chemically Dependent Patients at Risk for AIDS or Infected by HIV Virus.* Solicits names of chemical dependency programs that openly treat AIDS patients for referral purposes.

American Psychological Association   (National)
Scientific Affairs Office
1200 17th Street NW
Washington, DC 20036
(202) 955-7600

> Committee for Protection of Human Participants in Research and Committee on Gay Concerns issued *Statement on Ethical Issues in Psychological Research on AIDS.*

American Public Health Association   (National)
1015 15th Street NW
Washington, DC 20005
(202) 789-5600

> Promotes research in areas related to public health and communicable diseases. Publishes the *American Journal of Public Health, The Nation's Health*, a directory, and numerous books, manuals, and pamphlets.

American Red Cross   (National)
AIDS Education Office
1730 D Street NW
Washington, DC 20006
(202) 737-8300

Provides extensive information on varied aspects of AIDS including the safety of blood supplies, the AIDS antibody test, AIDS in the workplace, sexual practices and AIDS, AIDS and children, drug abuse, and homecare for the AIDS patient.

American Social Health Association (National)
260 Sheridan Avenue
Suite 307
Palo Alto, CA 94306
(800) 227-8922 (hotline)
(415) 321-5134

Produced a brochure series on social issues related to AIDS.

Arizona Step AIDS Project (Local)
736 East Slynn Main
Phoenix, AZ 85014
(602) 277-1929

Arkansas AIDS Foundation (Local)
P. O. Box 5007
Little Rock, AK 72225
(501) 224-4020

Association for Gay and Lesbian Issues in Counseling (National)
93 Ivy Street
Brookline, MA 02146
(617) 734-1958

Counselors and guidance workers concerned with lesbian and gay issues. Maintains a speakers' bureau.

Association for the Advancement of Health Education (National)
1900 Association Drive
Reston, VA 22091
(703) 476-3440

Comprised of professionals who are responsible for health education. Advances health education through programs and federal legislation. Encourages relationships between all health education and health service organizations.

Association of Gay and Lesbian Psychiatrists (National)
93 Ivy Street

Brookline, MA 02146
(617) 734-1958

> Promotes improved mental health services for homosexuals. Encourages research in areas related to homosexuality.

Association of Gay and Lesbian Psychologists   (National)
210 Fifth Avenue
New York, NY 10010

> Advocates the establishment of gay community service centers, gay counseling centers, and gay studies and programs.   Publishes the *Directory of Mental Health Practitioners* and *Directory of Psychologists Conducting Research on Lesbian/Gay Issues.*

Billings AIDS Support Network   (Local)
P. O. Box 1748
Billings, MT 59103
(406) 252-1212 (Hotline)

Bronx AIDS Community Service Project   (Local)
c/o South Bronx Development Organization
529 Courtland Avenue
Bronx, NY 10451

Brooklyn AIDS Community Service Program   (Local)
c/o Urban Resources Institute
22 Chapel Street
Brooklyn, NY 11201

Buffalo AIDS Task Force, Inc.   (Local)
220 Delaware Avenue
Suite 512
Buffalo, NY 14202
(716) 847-2441
(716) 847-2437

Center for Health Information   (National)
P. O. Box 4636
Foster City, CA 94404
(415) 345-6669

> Publishes literature related to AIDS.

Centers for Disease Control (CDC)   (National)
AIDS Activity Office
P. O. Box 5528
Building 3, Room 5B-1
1600 Clifton Road
Atlanta, GA 30307-0528
(404) 639-3311

> Publishes quarterly reports, a monthly newsletter, a bibliography, *Morbidity and Mortality Weekly Report (MMWR)*, and the *AIDS Weekly Surveillance Report.*

Colorado AIDS Project   (Local)
P. O. Box 18529
Denver, CO 80218
(303) 837-0166

Commission for Public Health   (National)
Suite 1217
1875 Connecticut Avenue NW
Washington, DC 20009
(202) 673-6888

Community AIDS Resource Association, Inc. (CARA)   (National)
P. O. Box 4534
Lafayette, IN 47903
(317) 742-9073
(317) 447-6811

> Free education and information services.

Community Health Information Resource Project (CHIRP)   (National)
Library and Information Services
West Suburban Hospital Medical Center
Erie at Austin
Oak Park, IL 60302
(312) 383-6200

Computerized AIDS Information Network (National)
1213 N. Highland Avenue
Hollywood, CA 90038
(213) 464-7400, ext. 277

Maintains a database on AIDS-related information.

Consumer Information Center   (National)
Department TD
Pueblo, CO 81009

Distributes free and inexpensive literature to the public.

D.C. AIDS Task Force   (Local)
Whitman Walker Clinic
2335 18th Street N W
Washington, DC 20009
(202) 332-5295
(202) 833-3234 (hotline Mon-Fri, 4-10 PM)

Extensive services that include testing, speakers, referral service, legal clinic, counseling, and bi-monthly newsletter.

FARO AIDS Action Council   (National)
111 S 1/2 Independence Avenue SE
Washington, DC 20003
(202) 547-3101

Formerly was the Federation of AIDS Related Organizations. Founded in 1982. Lobbies Congress on issues related to research funding for AIDS-related issues. Publishes the *AIDS Action Update*, a *Manual of Support Services for People With AIDS*, and *AIDS: A Political Handbook.*

Foundation for Health Education   (National)
P.O. Box 51537
New Orleans, LA 70151
(504) 244-6900

Fund for Human Dignity   (National)
666 Broadway, Fourth Floor
New York, NY 10012
(212) 529-1600
(800) 221-7044 (crisisline)

Operates a national clearinghouse of educational materials on gay/lesbian and AIDS-related issues. Maintains a crisisline and publishes *Fund Focus.* Affiliated with the National Gay and Lesbian Task Force.

Gay and Lesbian Alliance of Delaware   (Local)
P. O. Box 9218
Wilmington, DE 19809
(302) 764-2208
(800) 342-4012

Gay and Lesbian Press Association   (National)
P.O. Box A
Old Chelsea Station
New York, NY 10011
(212) 989-6622

Gay Men's Health Crisis   (National)
The AIDS Service and Education Foundation
Box 274, 132 West 24th Street
New York, NY 10011
(212) 807-7035 (hotline)
(212) 807-6572 (office)

Community-based organization dedicated to serving the needs of
people with AIDS, their friends, lovers, and families.

Gay Rights National Lobby   (National)
750 Seventh Street SE
Washington, DC 20013
(202) 546-1801

Involved in lobbying Congress on AIDS-related issues.

Good Samaritan Project   (National)
P. O. Box 10087
Kansas City, MO 64111-0087
(816) 452-2255

Haitian Coalition on AIDS   (Local)
Community Services
50 Court Street
Suite 1001
Brooklyn, NY 11201
(212) 855-7276

Health Education Resource Organization (HERO)   (National)
101 West Read Street, Suite 819
Baltimore, MD 21201
(301) 685-1180
(301) 947-AIDS
(301) 251-1164 (Metro DC area)
(800) 638-6252 (Maryland)
(301) 762-3385 (Montgomery County)
(301) 340-AIDS (Teen Hotline)

Non-profit community group formed in 1983. Provides accurate and confidential information and assistance to the public.

Health Related Services   (Local)
255 Eastern Parkway
Brooklyn, NY 11238
(212) 783-2676

Hispanic AIDS Forum   (National)
c/o APRED
853 Broadway
Suite 2007
New York, NY 10003
(212) 870-1902
(212) 870-1864

HLNL-Huey Lewis and the News   (National)
Physicians' AIDS Training Center
San Francisco General Hospital Medical Center
1001 Potrero Avenue
San Francisco, CA 94110

Program to train physicians how to deal with AIDS patients.

Homosexual Information Center   (National)
6758 Hollywood Boulevard, No. 208
Los Angeles, CA 90028
(213) 464-8431

Established in 1968, the Center provides general information on homosexuality as well as specialized, in-depth resources for scholars on topics such as AIDS. The resources of the Center are available to the media, legislative bodies, libraries, and the helping professions. Materials are available in five languages.

Hospice Association of America   (National)
210 Seventh Street SE
Suite 310
Washington, DC   20003
(202) 547-5263

Concerned with the care of AIDS patients.

Human Rights Campaign Fund   (National)
1012 14th Street NW
Suite 600
Washington, DC 20005
(202) 628-4160

Lobbies Congress for gay and lesbian civil rights and increased funding for AIDS research and treatment. Maintains a speakers' bureau and engages in fundraising activities.

Human Sexuality Program   (National)
Department of Health Education
School of Education, Health, Nursing and Arts Professions
New York University
239 Green Street, 6th Floor
New York, NY 10003
(212) 598-3926

School of scholars, researchers, teachers, and student devoted to the advancement and transmission of knowledge to society. Free pamphlet: *How to Talk to Your Children About AIDS.* Send self-addressed, stamped envelope.

Idaho AIDS Foundation   (Local)
P. O. Box 44123
Boise, ID 83711
(208) 345-2277

Illinois Alcoholism and Drug Dependence Association (IADDA)   (Local)
AIDS Project Office
c/o Interventions
1234 S. Michigan Avenue
Chicago, IL 60605
(312) 969-3168

Distributes a directory of AIDS services and provides referrrals.

Institute for the Protection of Lesbian and Gay Youth   (National)
110 E. 23rd Street, 10th Floor
New York, NY 10010
(212) 473-1113

> Provides service to gay and lesbian youth such as group and individual counseling and referral and education on human sexuality. Maintains a library for research on homosexuality.

International AIDS Prospective Epidemiology Network   (National)
155 N. Harbor Drive
Room 5103
Chicago, IL 60601
(312) 565-2103

> Provides a forum for health care workers, researchers and organizations to share data and information about AIDS; provides support to AIDS patients.

International Gay Information Center   (National)
P. O. Box 2
Village Station
New York, NY 10014
(718) 625-6463

> Purpose is to collect, preserve, document and disseminate information concerning the gay community. Extensive archival collection, tapes, newsclippings, and ephemera. Has an 8000-volume library and a speakers' bureau.

International Society on Infectious Diseases and Human Fertility
(National)
1430 Second Avenue
New York, NY 10021
(212) 774-5500

> Encourages the exchange of information among those involved in research on, and treatment of, sexually transmitted diseases.

International Union, AFL-CIO, CLC   (National)
1313 L Street NW
Washington, DC 20005
(202) 898-3200

> Provides informaton on AIDS in the workplace.

KS/AIDS Foundation (National)
3317 Montrose
Box 1155
Houston, TX 77006
(713) 524-2437

KS Research and Education Foundation (National)
54 Tenth Street
San Francisco, CA 94103
(415) 864-4376

Lambda Legal Defense and Education Fund (National)
666 Broadway
New York, NY 10012
(212) 944-9488

Offers legal services for the person with AIDS. Publishes the *AIDS Legal Guide: A Professional Resource on AIDS-Related Issues and Discrimination.*

Lesbian and Gay Caucus of the Democratic National Committee (National)
1742 Massachusetts Avenue SE
Washington, DC 20003
(202) 547-3104

Represents gay and lesbian concerns in the Democratic Party.

Lesbian Resource Center (National)
1212 E. Pine Street
Seattle, WA 98122
(206) 322-3965

Provides information on housing, employment, support groups, and social activities. Maintains lending library and research materials. Formerly **Gay Women's Alliance.**

Life Foundation (National)
320 Ward Avenue
Suite 104
Honolulu, HI 96814
(808) 924-2437

Lincoln Associates   (National)
P. O. Box 507
Madison, WI 53701

> Publishes *The Complete Reference Guide to AIDS*, which is a quarterly bibliography with five-year cumulations available.

Long Island Association for AIDS Care, Inc.   (Local)
P. O. Box 2859
1300 New York Avenue
Huntington Station, NY 11746
(516) 385-2451
(516) 385-2437

March of Dimes   (National)
1275 Mamaroneck Avenue
White Plains, NY 10605
(914) 428-7100

> Concerned with the effects of AIDS on children.   Publishes *Birth Defects Compendium.*

Metrolina AIDS Project   (Local)
P. O. Box 32662
Charlotte, NC 28232
(704) 333-2437
(704) 364-AIDS

Minority AIDS Project   (Local)
5882 West Rico Boulevard
Suite 210
Los Angeles, CA 90019
(800) 922-AIDS
(800) 222-SIDA (Spanish)
(213) 936-4949 (24-hour line)

Minority Task Force on AIDS   (Local)
c/o New York City Council of Churches
475 Riverside Drive
Room 456
New York, NY 10115
(212) 749-1214

Montana AIDS Project   (Local)
Department of Health and Environmental Science
Cogswell Building
Helena, MT 59620

Mothers of AIDS Patients (MAP)   (National)
3403 E. Street
San Diego, CA 92102
(619) 234-3432

National Academy of Sciences   (National)
Committee on a National Strategy for AIDS
Office of Public Affairs
2101 Constitution Avenue NW
Washington, DC 20418
(202) 334-2000

> Studies issues of vital importance to the nation. Publishes committee
> findings including the book, *Confronting AIDS.*

National AIDS Network   (National)
1012 14th Street NW
Suite 601
Washington, DC 20003
(202) 347-0390

> Created to link AIDS service providers by facilitating the exchange of
> ideas and information, by serving as a clearinghouse on AIDS
> programs and services, by providing technical assistance to member
> organizations, by assisting with the development of local and national
> education programs, and by coordinating fundraising efforts. Publishes
> the *Network News,* the *Monitor, AIDS Service Profiles,* and the *National
> AIDS Network Directory.*

National Association for Home Care   (National)
519 C Street NE
Washington, DC 20002
(202) 547-7424

> Disseminates information on homecare.

National Association of People With AIDS   (National)
P. O. Box 65472

Washington, DC 20035
(202) 483-7979
(202) 797-3708

Clearinghouse for services and information to people with AIDS.

National Association of Public Hospitals   (National)
1426 21st Street NW
Suite 10
Washington, DC 20036
(202) 861-0434

Conducted a detailed survey on the hospital care to patients with AIDS in major U.S. public and private teaching institutions in 1985. Published results in the September 11, 1987 issue of *JAMA, Journal of the American Medical Association.*

National Association of Social Workers   (National)
National Committee on Lesbian and Gay Issues
7981 Eastern Avenue
Silver Spring, MD 20910
(301) 565-0333
            or
110 West 86th Street
New York, NY 10024
(212) 799-3298

National Coalition of Black Lesbians and Gays   (National)
1716 Florida Avenue NW
Washington, DC 20009
(202) 265-7117

National Coalition of Gay Sexually Transmitted Disease Services   (National)
P. O. Box 239
Milwaukee, WI 53201
(414) 277-7671

Disseminates information, provides speakers, and publishes a bi-monthly newsletter and pamphlets with guidelines and recommendations for healthy sexual activity for the medical, scientific, and gay communities. Gay clinics and AIDS service organizations throughout the U.S. belong to the Coalition, which maintains a liaison with the Centers for Disease Control.

National Council of Churches of Christ   (National)
AIDS Task Force
475 Riverside Drive
Room 573
New York, NY 10115
(212) 870-2421
(212) 870-2385

National Education Association   (National)
1201 16th Street NW
Washington, DC 20036
(202) 833-4000

> Endorses AIDS education in the public schools and produces information about AIDS in the classroom.

National Gay and Lesbian Task Force   (National)
80 Fifth Avenue
Suite 1601
New York, NY 10011
(800) 221-7044 (hotline)
(212) 807-6016 (in NY from 3-9 PM)
   or
2335 18th Street NW
Washington, DC 20009
(202) 332-6483

> Serves as a clearinghouse of information for the general public, persons with AIDS and their families, and health care workers. Does extensive lobbying on aids-related issues. Publishes the *Task Force Report*, a bi-monthly newsletter, and various AIDS updates.

National Gay Health Education Foundation   (National)
P. O. Box 784
New York, NY 10036
(212) 563-6313

> Founded in 1980 to coordinate educational activities, develop programs, and encourage research in gay and lesbian health care issues. Publishes a directory of AIDS services and the annual *National Gay Health Directory*.

National Gay Rights Advocates   (National)
540 Castro Street
San Francisco, CA 94114
(415) 863-3624

Provides legal services.

National Hemophilia Association (National)
110 Greene Street
Room 406
New York, NY 10012
(212) 563-0211
(212) 682-5510 (hotline Mon-Fri 9 AM-5 PM)

>Provides information for hemophiliacs and their physicians. Maintains *The Hemophilia Information Exchange.*

National League for Nursing (National)
Ten Columbus Circle
New York, NY 10019
(212) 582-1022

>Deals with issues related to nursing the AIDS patient and homecare of the AIDS patient.

National Lesbian and Gay Health Foundation (National)
P. O. Box 65472
Washington, DC 20035
(202) 797-3708

>Promotes lesbian/gay health care issues and concerns, serves as a clearinghouse, and conducts annual conferences on lesbian/gay studies. Publishes an annual directory of lesbian/gay health services.

New Orleans AIDS Task Force (Local)
P. O. Box 2616
New Orleans, LA 70116
(504) 891-3732

>Maintains a speakers' bureau; provides referrals for medical and legal services; has a library of literature, slides, videotapes, and other educational material; conducts community educational programs; and has a staff of trained volunteers.

Northwest AIDS Foundation (Local)
P. O. Box 3449
Seattle, WA 98114
(206) 527-8770 or
(206) 622-9650

People With AIDS Coalition   (National)
263A West 19th Street
Room 125
New York, NY 10011
(212) 627-1810

Maintains a speakers' bureau, distributes literature, provides support services and referrals to appropriate resource organizations, conducts public forums, and maintains a drop-in lounge.   Publishes *PWA Coalition Newsline.*

Philadelphia AIDS Task Force   (Local)
P. O. Box 7259
Philadelphia, PA 19101
(215) 232-8055

Planned Parenthood Federation of America   (National)
810 Seventh Avenue
New York, NY 10019
(212) 541-7800

Develops information, education, and training programs to increase knowledge about human sexual health.

Project Inform   (National)
25 Taylor Street
Suite 618
San Francisco, CA 94102
(800) 822-7422 (National)
(800) 334-7422 (California)
(415) 928-0293 (Local)

This information service is sponsored by the Documentation of AIDS Issues and Research Foundation, Inc. (DAIR), a non-profit foundation which studies and distributes information on drug effectiveness, but does not recommend or endorse treatment modalities.

Rhode Island Project AIDS   (Local)
22 Hayes Street
Room 124
Providence, RI 02903
(401) 277-6502

St. Francis Center   (Local)
2201 P Street NW
Washington, DC 20037
(202) 234-5613

Provides grief and bereavement counseling.

St. Louis Effort for Aids   (Local)
1120 Dolman
St. Louis, MO 63104
(314) 421-3914

Salt Lake AIDS Foundation   (Local)
3450 Highland Drive #102
Salt Lake City, UT 84106
(801) 466-9976

San Diego AIDS Project   (Local)
4304 Third Avenue
P. O. Box 81082
San Diego, CA 92138
(619) 543-0300

San Francisco AIDS Foundation   (National)
25 Van Ness Street
San Francisco, CA 94102
(415) 864-4376 (office)
(415) 863-AIDS (hotline in San Francisco)
(800) FOR-AIDS (hotline for outside of San Francisco)

Established in 1982, this organization provides extensive literature, information, and referral services. Maintains a speakers' bureau and a list of AIDS-sensitive health providers.

Shanti Project of San Francisco   (Local)
525 Howard Street
San Francisco, CA 94105
(415) 777-CARE

A psychosocial program dealing with housing for AIDS patients. Coordinates a peer counseling service and a home help volunteer program.

Shreveport GLAD   (Local)
P. O. Box 4523
Shreveport, LA 71104
(318) 222-4523

Provides anonymous HIV testing and phone counseling.

SIECUS (Sex Information and Education Council of the U.S.)   (National)
New York University
32 Washington Place, 5th Floor
New York, NY 10003
(212) 673-3850

This is a private, nonprofit, educational organization that was established in 1964 to promote healthy sexuality. Provides information and education on sexual matters to the public through a clearinghouse and resource center. Membership fee is $60. The bi-monthly journal, *The SIECUS Report*, is included in membership.

Southern Tier AIDS Program, Inc.   (Local)
65 Broad Street
Johnson City, NY 13790
(607) 798-1706
(607) 723-6520 (hotline)

Coordinates support services for people impacted by AIDS and provides education on AIDS through a speakers' bureau, hotline, support groups, buddy program, and fundraising.

United Community Services   (Local)
51 West Warren Avenue
Detroit, MI 48201
(313) 833-0622

U.S. Conference of Local Health Officers   (National)
1620 Eye Street NW
Washington, DC 20006
(202) 293-7330

Founded in 1960, this organization of local health departments seeks to make timely and appropriate information on AIDS available to mayors and local health officials.

U.S. Conference of Mayors   (National)
1620 I Street NW

Fourth Floor
Washington, DC 20006
(202) 293-7330

Publishes a directory of AIDS-related services.

Vermont Cares   (Local)
P. O. Box 1125
Montpelier, VT 05602

Wellness Networks, Inc.   (National)
P. O. Box 1046
Royal Oak, MI 48068
(800) 482-2404, ext. 3582 (in Michigan)
(800) 521-7946, ext. 3582 (outside of Michigan)
(313) 876-3582 (in Detroit)

Dedicated to the promotion of positive health practices and lifestyles through information and referrals, this non-profit corporation solicits volunteer help.

Women's AIDS Network   (National)
c/o San Francisco AIDS Foundation
25 Van Ness Street
San Francisco, CA 94102

Serves as a clearinghouse and information network for women doing AIDS-related work. Seeks to find resources to deal with issues relating to women.

World Health Organization Collaborating Centre on AIDS   (National)
c/o Centers for Disease Control
1600 Clifton Road NE
Atlanta, GA 30333
(404) 329-3311

Chartered by the WHO to conduct research and public health programs on AIDS; provides instruction to health workers and laboratory technicians, maintains a speakers' bureau, and compiles statistics.

World Hemophilia AIDS Center   (National)
2400 S. Flower Street
Los Angeles, CA 90007
(213) 742-1357

Serves as a clearinghouse and surveillance center for AIDS in hemophilia patients. Publishes the quarterly *Hemophilia World.*

Health Departments

The departments of health are a major link to the many resources available within each state. The range of services are as diversified as the department names themselves. Often the office that deals with AIDS-related issues has the word "AIDS" in its title, such as the "AIDS Program" of Missouri or the "Special Office on AIDS Prevention" of Michigan. Several states have multiple offices and telephone numbers for multiple purposes. Some offices handle all the aspects of public information related to AIDS such as phone and mail requests for information, and educational development. A separate office may handle statistical data or information for the health professional. Most states accept phone requests and provide such information as referrals to statewide test sites, locations of counseling services, general support services for AIDS/ARC patients, legal assistance, crisis intervention services, and willing health care providers. Many state departments maintain hotlines and some have a speakers' bureau of personnel available to make presentations to both the general public and to health professionals. Some offices also provide curriculum outlines and lesson plans to assist educators in the classroom. Most departments distribute literature from the U.S. Public Health Service and the American Red Cross as well as pamphlets and posters that have been devised internally. Core directories of statewide services related to AIDS are often available upon request.

ALABAMA
Sexually Transmitted Disease Branch
Department of Public Health
State Office Building
Room 252
501 Dexter Avenue
Montgomery, AL 36130-1701
(205) 261-5017

ALASKA
Division of Public Health
Department of Health and Social Services

Pouch H-06
Juneau, AK 99811
(907) 465-3090

ARIZONA
AIDS Project
Office of Health Promotion and Education
Arizona Department of Health Services
3008 North 3rd Street
Phoenix, AZ 85012
(602) 230-5838

Division of Disease Control Services
Arizona Department of Health Services
431 North 24th Street
Phoenix, AZ 85088
(602) 255-1280

ARKANSAS
Division of Communicable Diseases
Arkansas State Department of Health
4815 West Markham, Room 473
Little Rock, AR 72201
(800) 445-7720

CALIFORNIA
Office of AIDS
Department of Health Services
State of California
P. O. Box 160146
714/744 P Street
Sacramento, CA 95814
(916) 445-0553

COLORADO
STD/AIDS Program
Colorado Department of Health
4210 East 11th Avenue
Denver, CO 80220
(303) 320-8333
(303) 331-8305 (24 hour recording)

CONNECTICUT
AIDS Program
Department of Health Services
State of Connecticut
150 Washington Street
Hartford, CT 06106
(203) 566-1157
(203) 566-4800

DELAWARE
AIDS Program Office
Bureau of Disease Control
Division of Public Health
Department of Health and Social Services
State of Delaware
Building G
3000 Newport Gap Pike
Wilmington, DE 19808
(302) 995-8422

DISTRICT OF COLUMBIA
Department of Human Services
Commission of Public Health
1875 Connecticut Avenue NW
Washington, DC 20009

FLORIDA
Department of Health
1317 Winewood Boulevard
Tallahassee, FL 32301
(904) 488-2945

Health Crisis Network
P.O. Box 42-1280
Miami, FL 33242-1280
(305) 326-8833
(305) 634-4636

GEORGIA
Division of Public Health
Georgia Department of Human Resources
47 Trinity Avenue SW
Atlanta, GA 30334
(800) 342-7514

HAWAII
Department of Health
1250 Punchbowl Street
Honolulu, HI 96801
(808) 735-5303

IDAHO
AIDS Health Educator
Division of Health
Department of Health and Welfare
450 West State Street
Boise, ID 83720
(208) 334-5944

ILLINOIS
Infectious Disease - AIDS
Illinois Department of Public Health
100 West Randolph 6-600
Chicago, IL 60601
(312) 917-3880
(800) AID-AIDS
(312) 744-4305

Infectious Disease
Illinois Department of Public Health
535 West Jefferson
Springfield, IL 62761
(217) 782-2016

INDIANA
AIDS Activity Office
Indiana State Board of Health
P. O. Box 1964
1330 West Michigan Street
Indianapolis, IN 46206-1964
(317) 633-8406
(317) 633-8051

IOWA
Sexually Transmitted Disease Section
Division of Disease Prevention - 00
Iowa Department of Public Health
Lucas State Office Building

Des Moines, IA 50319-0075
(800) 445-AIDS (24 hour line)
(800) 532-3301 (Mon - Fri 8 a.m. - 4:30 p.m.)

KANSAS

Bureau of Community Health
Kansas Department of Health and Environment
Landon State Office Building
Topeka, KA 66620-0001
(913) 296-5585
(913) 296-1216

KENTUCKY

STD Control Program
Cabinet for Human Resources
Department of Health Services
Commonwealth of Kentucky
275 East Main Street
Frankfort, KY 40621-0001
(502) 564-4804

LOUISIANA

Department of Health and Human Resources
755 Riverside, North
Baton Rouge, LA 70802
(504) 342-6711

MAINE

Office on AIDS
STD Control Program
Bureau of Health
Department of Human Services
State House Station 11
Augusta, ME 04333
(207) 289-3747

MARYLAND

Division of Health
Maryland Department of Health & Mental Hygiene
201 W. Preston Street
Baltimore, MD 21201
(301) 383-6196

MASSACHUSETTS
Office of Health Resources
Massachusetts Department of Public Health
150 Tremont Street, Ninth Floor
Boston, MA 02111
(617) 727-0368

AIDS Program/Alternative Test Site Program
State Laboratory Institute
Massachusetts Department of Public Health
305 South Street
Jamaica Plain, MA 02130
(617) 727-9080 -- for HIV testing information
(617) 522-3700, ext. 472. -- for health care providers
(617) 522-3700, ex. 476 -- for case reporting and statistics

MICHIGAN
Special Office on AIDS Prevention
Center for Health Promotion
Michigan Department of Public Health
3500 N. Logan Street
P. O. Box 30035
Lansing, MI 48909
(517) 335-8371

MINNESOTA
Department of Health
717 Delaware Street SE
Minneapolis, MN 55440
(612) 870-0700
(800) 752-4281

MISSISSIPPI
AIDS Information
Mississippi State Department of Health
Jackson, MI 39215-1700
(601) 960-7725
(800) 826-2961 (14 hrs. daily)

MISSOURI
AIDS Program
Department of Health
State of Missouri
P. O. Box 570

1730 East Elm
Jefferson City, MO 65102-0570
(314) 751-6438

MONTANA
Department of Health and Environmental Sciences
Cogswell Building
Helena, MT 59620
(406) 444-4740

NEBRASKA
AIDS Program
Department of Health
State of Nebraska
301 Centennial Mall South
P. O. Box 95007
Lincoln, NE 68509
(402) 471-2937

NEVADA
Division of Health
Department of Human Resources
505 E. King Street
Carson City, NV 89710
(702) 885-4988

NEW HAMPSHIRE
Division of Public Health Services
Department of Health and Welfare
Hazen Drive
Concord, NH 03301
(603) 271-4487

NEW JERSEY
AIDS Office
New Jersey Department of Health
Room 100 CN 360
Trenton, NJ 08625
(800) 624-2377 (within NJ)
(800) 367-6543 (outside of NJ)
Inquiries for information accepted only by mail.

NEW MEXICO
Division of Health Services
New Mexico Department of Health and Environment
725 St. Michael's Drive
Santa Fe, NM 87504
(505) 984-0030

NEW YORK
Center for Community Health
Division of Epidemiology
Bureau of Communicable Disease Control
New York State Department of Health
Empire State Plaza
Corning Tower
Albany, NY 12237
(518) 474-3186
(518) 473-0641
(212) 340-3388

Division of Health Promotion
New York City Department of Health
125 Worth Street, Box 46
New York, NY 10013
(212) 566-7103
(718) 485-8111

NORTH CAROLINA
Division of Health Services
Department of Human Resources
225 North McDowell Street
Raleigh, NC 27603
(919) 733-7301

NORTH DAKOTA
Department of Health
State Capitol
Bismarck, ND 58505
(701) 224-2378
(800) 472-2180

OHIO
The AIDS Unit
Ohio Department of Health
246 N. High Street

P. O. Box 118
Columbus, OH 43266-0118
(614) 466-3543

OKLAHOMA
Sexually Transmitted Disease Division
Oklahoma State Department of Health
1000 Northeast 10th Street
P. O. Box 53551
Oklahoma City, OK 73152
(405) 271-4061

OREGON
Divison of Health
Department of Human Resources
1400 S. W. 5th Avenue
Portland, OR 97201
(503) 229-5792

PENNSYLVANIA
Division of Health Promotion
Pennsylvania State Department of Health
Room 614
Health and Welfare Building
P. O. Box 90
Harrisburg, PA 17108
(800) 692-7254
(717) 737-5349 (Mon - Fri 7:30 a.m. - 4:30 p.m.)

RHODE ISLAND
Department of Health
State of Rhode Island and Providence Plantations
Cannon Building
75 Davis Street
Providence, RI 02908
(401) 277-2362

SOUTH CAROLINA
Office of Health Protection
Department of Health and Environmental Control
2600 Bull Street
Columbia, SC 29201
(803) 734-5482

SOUTH DAKOTA
Department of Health
523 East Capitol
Pierre, SD 57501
(605) 773-3357

TENNESSEE
AIDS Program
Bureau of Health Services
Tennessee Department of Health and Environment
One Hundred 9th Avenue, North
Nashville, TN 37219-5405
(615) 741-7387

TEXAS
Public Health Promotion Division
Texas Department of Health
1100 West 49th Street
Austin, TX 78756-3199
(512) 458-7225 (STD Control Division)
(512) 458-7405 (Public Health Promotion Division)
(512) 458-7504 (AIDS Surveillance Program)

UTAH
AIDS Program
Bureau of Epidemiology
Division of Community Health Services
U⁺⁻h Department of Health
P. ᴜ. Box 16660
288 North 1460 West
Salt Lake City, UT 84116-0660
(801) 538-6191

VERMONT
AIDS Educator
Department of Epidemiology
60 Main Street
Burlington, VT 05401
(802) 863-7240

VIRGINIA
STD Control
Virginia State Health Department
109 Governor Street

Richmond, VA 23219
(800) 533-4148 (8:30 a.m. - 5:00 p.m.)
(804) 225-4844
(804) 786-0877

WASHINGTON (State)
AIDS Program
Department of Social and Health Services
Airdustrial Park
Building 14, LP-13
Olympia, WA 98504
(206) 753-3460

Washington State AIDS Surveillance Unit
Department of Social and Health Services
1610 N. E. 150th Street
Seattle, WA 98155
(206) 361-2914

WEST VIRGINIA
AIDS Health Educator
Division of Epidemiology
Department of Health
Capitol Complex 3
Charleston, WV 25305
(304) 348-5358

WISCONSIN
Section of Acute and Communicable Disease Epidemiology
Division of Health
Wisconsin Department of Health and Social Services
1 West Wilson Street
P. O. Box 309
Madison, WI 53701
(608) 267-5287

WYOMING
AIDS Program Coordinator
Department of Health and Social Services
Hathaway Building
Cheyenne, WY 82002
(307) 777-7953
(307) 237-7833

Research Institutions, Grant Funding Sources, and Federal Agencies

The majority of research funding is supplied by the Federal Government. However, several major funding sources or organizations that coordinate grant monies have emerged in the private sector. The following is a listing of resources that can be tapped for grant funding, agencies that conduct research specific to AIDS, and federal agencies that both provide funds as well as conduct research. Additional federal agencies are identified that coordinate specific services for the AIDS patient nationwide. Several sources exist that continually provide updated information related to research and grant funding. These include the *AmFar Directory of Experimental Treatments for AIDS & ARC* and the *National Institutes of Health Guide for Grants and Contracts*.

RESEARCH INSTITUTIONS

Abbott Laboratories
Public Affairs, Department 383P
Route 137
Abbott Park
Chicago, IL 60064
(312) 937-6100

Publishes a public service pamphlet for general distribution and conducts research on AIDS treatment.

Ackerman Institute for Family Therapy
149 East 78th Street
New York, NY 10021
(212) 879-4900

Conducts research on AIDS and ARC. Provides training and sponsors conferences and workshops for professionals in the psychosocial fields.

Addiction Research and Treatment Corporation
22 Chapel Street
Brooklyn, NY 11201
(718) 834-5300

> Researches the relationship of drug and alcohol addiction to sexual practices and exposure to the AIDS virus.

Army Medical Research Institute of Infectious Diseases
Department of the Army
Office of the Surgeon General of the Army
Army Medical Research and Development Command
Building 1425, SGRD UIA-L
Fort Detrick
Frederick, MD 21701
(301) 663-2720 (Medical Library)

Baylor University College of Medicine
Center for Allergy and Immunological Disorders
1200 Moursund Avenue
Houston, TX 77030
(713) 791-4219
(713) 790-4768 (General Clinical Research Center)
(713) 790-4443 (Virus Research Center)

Baylor University College of Medicine
Center for Ethics, Medicine, and Public Issues
1200 Moursund Avenue
Houston, TX 77030
(713) 799-6290

> Studies the ethical problems in the care of AIDS patients.

Baylor University College of Medicine
Virus Research Center
1200 Moursund Avenue
Houston, TX 77030
(713) 799-4443

> Involved in AIDS viral studies.

Bio-Research Institute, Inc.
9 Commercial Avenue
Cambridge, MA 02141

Cancer Research Institute (CRI)
New England Deaconess Hospital
185 Pilgrim
Boston, MA 02215
(617) 732-8016

> Affiliated with Harvard University School of Medicine. Conducts research on AIDS.

Center for Blood Research
800 Huntington Avenue
Boston, MA 02115
(617) 731-6470

Center for Interdisciplinary Research in Immunology and Disease (CIRID)
c/o Department of Microbiology and Immunology
UCLA School of Medicine
Factor Building, Room 12-248
Los Angeles, CA 90024
(213) 825-1510

> Conducts research on AIDS. Results published in the *NIAID Annual Report*, the *AIDS Medical Update*, and the *AIDS Reference Guide for Medical Professionals*. Maintains a library on immunology.

Centers for Disease Control (CDC)
AIDS Activity
P. O. Box 5528
Building 3, Room 5B-1
1600 Clifton Road
Atlanta, GA 30307-0528
(404) 874-7151

> Publishes quarterly reports, a monthly newsletter, a bibliography, *Morbidity and Mortality Weekly Report (MMWR)*, and the *AIDS Weekly Surveillance Report.*

Documentation of AIDS Issues and Research Foundation (DAIR)
25 Taylor Street, Suite 618
San Francisco, CA 94102
(415) 928-0293

> Non-profit foundation; sponsors Project Inform -- information service.

Georgetown University
School of Medicine
International Center for Interdisciplinary Studies of Immunology at
    Georgetown
3800 Reservoir Road NW
Washington, DC 20007
(202) 625-7437

Research interests in the fields of infectious diseases and disorders of
immune regulation.

Gorgas Memorial Laboratory
P. O. Box 935, APO
Miami, FL 34002
(Panama) 25-4366

Studies AIDS in Panama and provides statistical consultation to
medical professionals.

**Independent Citizens Research Foundation for Study of Degenerative
    Diseases, Inc.**
P. O. Box 97
Ardsley, NY 10502
(914) 478-1862

Studies the causes and treatment of AIDS. Publishes bulletins and
newsletters. Maintains a library.

Institute for Immunological Disorders
7407 North Freeway
Houston, TX 77076
(713) 691-3531

Conducts experimental studies on the treatment of AIDS and ARC
and the antiviral drug ribavirin.

Institute of Cancer Research
710 Standford Building
2200 Webster Street
San Francisco, CA 94115
(415) 561-1688

As a part of the Medical Research Institute of San Francisco, conducts
clinical research on AIDS.

Kaiser Foundation Research Institute
3505 Broadway
Suite 1112
Oakland, CA 94611
(415) 428-6332

Conducts clinical trials dealing with AIDS.

Kuzell Institute for Arthritis and Infectious Diseases
Medical Research Institute of San Francisco
2200 Webster Street, R305
San Francisco, CA 94115
(415) 561-1734

Basic and applied research with AIDS.

Mariposa Education and Research Foundation, Inc.
P. O. Box 36B35
Los Angeles, CA 90036
(818) 704-4812

Conducts research on the prevention of AIDS.

Maryland Medical Research Institute
600 Windhurst Avenue
Baltimore, MD 21210
(301) 435-4200

Data gathering, analysis, and design for large-scale clinical trials in AIDS. Publishes the quarterly *Controlled Clinical Trials* and conducts seminars in association with the University of Maryland.

Massachusetts General Hospital
32 Fruit Street
Boston, MA 02114
(617) 726-2000

National Cancer Institute
NIH Building 10
9000 Rockville Pike
Bethesda, MD 20892

(301) 496-5461 (Immunology Branch)
(301) 496-4916 (Medicine Branch)
(301) 496-6007 (Tumor Cell Biology Laboratory)

Investigates the immunosuppressive events associated with and leading to AIDS.

National Institutes of Health and World Health Organization Collaborating Center for Reference and Research in Simian Viruses
P. O. Box 28147
San Antonio, TX 78284
(512) 674-1410

Conducts studies on AIDS and Simian Acquired Immunodeficiency Syndrome in nonhuman primates.

New Orleans AIDS Research Consortium
c/o Paul Balson, MD
Department of Psychiatry
Louisiana State University
1542 Tulane Avenue
New Orleans, LA 70112

Consortium of scientists, educators, and health care professionals. Focus on mental health aspects of AIDS.

New York State Center for Assessing Health Services
Health Sciences Center, 4L-215
Stony Brook, NY 11794
(516) 444-2101

Studies the cost of treating patients with AIDS.
Publishes two bi-monthly publications: *New Technology Abstracts* and *Current Assessments.*

New York University
Kaplan Cancer Center
550 First Avenue
New York, NY 10016
(212) 340-5349

Conducts cancer research and its relation to AIDS and Kaposi's sarcoma. Publishes the *Kaplan Center Newsletter.* Sponsors an annual seminar.

New York University
Laboratory for Experimental Medicine and Surgery in Primates
5500 First Avenue
New York, NY 10016
(212) 340-6626

Serves as a cooperative research and educational facility for the investigation of AIDS using chimpanzees.

Ohio State University
Infectious Diseases Research Laboratories
410 West 10th Avenue
Columbus, OH 43210
(614) 421-8640

Researches the pathology, therapy, and prophylaxis of infectious diseases including AIDS.

Pennsylvania State University
Milton S. Hershey Medical Center
Division of Hematology
School of Medicine
P. O. Box 850
Hershey, PA 17033
(717) 531-8399

Research on hemophilias and AIDS.

Pennsylvania State University
Milton S. Hershey Medical Center
Department of Microbiology
School of Medicine
P. O. Box 850
Hershey, PA 17033
(717) 531-8258

Conducts research on the HTLV-III virus.

Pitt Men's Study
University of Pittsburgh
Department of Infectious Diseases and Microbiology
P. O. Box 7319
Pittsburgh, PA 15213
(412) 624-20008

Study funded by NIH. Open to all men who have had homosexual contact in the last five years. Following the natural history of AIDS in homosexual and bisexual men.

Tulane University
School of Medicine
Clinical Immunology Section
1700 Perdido Street, Third Floor
New Orleans, LA 70112
(504) 588-5578

Research on immune deficiencies and autoimmune disorders, especially mechanisms of acquired immune deficiency syndrome.

University of California, Los Angeles
UCLA AIDS Clinical Research Center
VAMC West Los Angeles
691/W111P
Los Angeles, CA 90073
(213) 206-6414

Conducts clinical research trials on AIDS and AIDS-related disease. Maintains a blood/serum and a tissue/lymph node bank of specimens to other AIDS researchers. Publishes *UCLA AIDS Medical Update* and *UCLA AIDS Nursing Update.*

University of California Los Angeles Medical Center
10833 LeConte Avenue
Los Angeles, CA 90024
(213) 825-9111

University of California, San Francisco
AIDS Clinical Research Center
4150 Clement Street
San Francisco, CA 94121
(415) 221-4810

Involved with epidemiological studies, immunological investigations, protocol development, data collection and analysis, and educational programs. Is comprised of the AIDS treatment units in the three University of California, San Francisco teaching hospitals.

University of California, San Francisco
General Clinical Research Center (GCRC)
San Francisco General Hospital

1001 Potrero Avenue
Building 100, Ward 18
San Francisco, CA 94110
(415) 285-2900

Researches adrenal defects in AIDS.

University of California, San Francisco
Institute for Health Policy Studies
1326 Third Avenue
San Francisco, CA 94143
(415) 476-4921

Conducts studies on the cost of AIDS.

University of California San Francisco Hospitals and Clinics
AIDS Clinical Research Center
905 Parnassus Avenue
San Francisco, CA 94143
(415) 666-1407

Researches AIDS and Kaposi sarcoma and maintains a tissue bank with patient information for cooperative investigations.

University of Colorado -- Denver
School of Medicine
Allergy and Immunology Center
4700 E. 9th Street
Denver, CO 80262
(303) 394-7601

Researches immune deficiencies and autoimmune disorders.

University of Pennsylvania
Comparative Leukemia Unit
New Bolton Center
382 West Street Road
Kennett Square, PA 19348
(215) 444-5800

Studies include bovine leukemia virus (BLV) and its relationship to human T-cell lymphotropic virus type one (HTLV-1) and the AIDS virus.

University of Southern California
Hematology Research Laboratory
2025 Zonal Avenue
Los Angeles, CA 90033
(213) 224-7224

Clinical research on AIDS.

GRANT FUNDING SOURCES

AIDS Medical Foundation
10 East 13th Street
New York, NY 10003
(212) 206-0670

Founded in 1983 to raise funds for research.

Alcohol, Drug Abuse, and Mental Health Administration
5600 Fishers Lane
Parklawn Building
Rockville, MD 20857
(301) 443-6697

Provides support to establish AIDS Research Centers on the mental
health and drug abuse aspects of AIDS, ARC, and HTLV-III infection.

American Foundation for AIDS Research
40 West 57th Street
New York, NY 10019
(212) 588-1454

National group formed to conduct and support biomedical research
and public education to bring about the end of the AIDS epidemic.
Elizabeth Taylor is the national chairman.

Centers for Disease Control (CDC)
Grants Management Office
Department of Health and Human Services
255 E. Paces Ferry Road NE
Room 321
Atlanta, GA 30305
(404) 262-6575

Sponsors Acquired Immunodeficiency Syndrome (AIDS) Project Grants to fund programs that would conduct epidemiological studies, health education projects, and prevention activities.

Flintridge Foundation
1100 El Centro Street, Suite 103
South Pasadena, CA 91030
(818) 799-4178

Provides support for medical and scientific research on AIDS education.

Freed Foundation, Inc.
1200 Eton Court NW
Washington, DC 20007
(202) 296-6406

Grants for AIDS research for organizations primarily in the Washington, DC and New Jersey areas.

Health Resources and Services Administration
Office of AIDS Service Programs
Room 9-21
5600 Fishers Lane
Rockville, MD 20657
(301) 443-6745

Grants on educational and training centers and AIDS service projects.

National AIDS Network
1012 14th Street NW
Suite 601
Washington, DC 20005
(202) 347-0390

Provides grants to AIDS agencies as well as advertises granting opportunities in the semi-monthly publication, *Network News*.

National Cancer Institute
Research Contracts Branch
Treatment Contracts Section
Blair Building, Room 224
Bethesda, MD 20892-4200

Contracts with organizations to study the pharmacological and toxicology aspects of anti-AIDS agents.

National Heart, Lung, and Blood Institute
Blood Resources Branch
Contracts Section
Federal Building, Room 5C14
Bethesda, MD 20892-4200

Supports the development of new tests to identify the HTLV-III virus in blood donors.

National Institute on Alcohol Abuse and Alcoholism
National Centers and Special Programs Branch
Division of Extramural Research
5600 Fishers Lane
Parklawn Building, Room 14C20
Rockville, MD 20857
(301) 443-1273

Funds Alcohol Aspects of AIDS Research Grants to research the epidemiology, possible underlying mechanisms, and other possible correlations of AIDS and alcohol.

National Institute of Allergy and Infectious Diseases
AIDS Program Officer
Clinical Studies Branch
Building 31, Room 7A49
Bethesda, MD 20892-4200
(301) 496-5893

Sponsors Acquired Immunodeficiency Syndrome (AIDS) Research Grants to fund studies on the development of vaccines, treatment trials, in vitro testing and animal research, and epidemiology, pathogenesis, and treatment of AIDS.

National Institute of Allergy and Infectious Diseases
Clinical and Epidemiological Studies Branch
5333 Westbard Avenue
Room 707
Bethesda, MD 20892-4200

Provides funding for research facilities to determine an effective treatment regimen for AIDS infection and/or related opportunistic diseases.

National Institute of Mental Health
5600 Fishers Lane
Parklawn Building
Room 11C06
Rockville, MD 20857
(301) 443-3463

Publishes the booklet, *Coping With AIDS*, and provides grant funding on the psychological aspects of AIDS.

National Institute on Drug Abuse
5600 Fishers Lane
Parklawn Building, Room 10-16
Rockville, MD 20857

Supports research on AIDS and ARC among drug abusers.

National Institutes of Health
AIDS Drug Selection Committee
9000 Rockville Pike
Building 31, Room 3A49
Bethesda, MD 20892-4200

Sponsors AIDS Treatments Development Research Grants to facilitate the development and testing of possible treatments for AIDS.

National Institutes of Health
Division of Research Grants
Westwood Building
5333 Westbard Avenue
Bethesda, MD 20205
(301) 496-7179

National Institutes of Health
Division of Research Resources
9000 Rockville Pike
Bethesda, MD 20205
(301) 496-5131 (Grants and contracts)

National Institutes of Health
Division of Research Services
9000 Rockville Pike

Bethesda, MD 20205
(301) 496-5795 (Public inquiries)

Robert Wood Johnson Foundation
AIDS Health Services Program
P. O. Box 2316
Forrestal Center
Princeton, NJ 08543-2316
(609) 452-8701

> Grants available for healthcare agencies to explore ways to provide more humane care to AIDS patients.

STAMP OUT AIDS
240 West 44th Street
New York, NY 10036

> Provides grant funding for direct AIDS victim care through the sale of special stamps.

OTHER FEDERAL SOURCES OF INFORMATION

Human Development Services
Office of Public Affairs
200 Independence Avenue SW
Washington, DC 20201
(202) 472-7257

National Health Information Clearinghouse
Office of Disease Prevention and Health
Public Health Service
P. O. Box 1133
Washington, DC 20013
(800) 336-4797

National Institute of Allergy and Infectious Diseases
Office of Research Reporting and Public Response
9000 Rockville Pike
Building 31, Room 7A32
National Institutes of Health
Bethesda, MD 20892
(301) 496-5717

Office of Technology Assessment
600 Pennsylvania Avenue SE
Washington, DC 20510
(202) 226-2070

U.S. Environmental Protection Agency
Disinfectants Branch
Office of Pesticides
401 M. Street SW
Washington, DC 20460

> Provides information on germicides and disinfectants to use in sterilization of materials.

U.S. Food and Drug Administration
Blood and Blood Products Division
Room 220, NIH Building 29
Bethesda, MD 21235
(301) 496-4396

> Responsible for blood donor policy and licensing of blood tests.

U.S. House of Representatives
Select Committee on Children, Youth, and Families
385 House Office Building
Annex 2
Washington, DC 20515
(202) 226-7692

> Published findings of a hearing on the increased incidence of babies born with AIDS, the care of AIDS infected children, and prevention efforts.

U.S. Public Health Service
Public Affairs Office
Hubert H. Humphrey Building, Room 725-H
200 Independence Avenue, SW
Washington, DC 20201
(202) 245-6867
(800) 342-2437 (Hotline with a taped message)

> Provides information to the public on the prevention of AIDS.

U.S. Social Security Administration
900 Altmeyer Building
Baltimore, MD 21235
(301) 564-3120

Administers financial benefits for persons with AIDS.

Hotlines

Hotlines are usually synonomous with referral services or information clearinghouses, but also can be one aspect of an organization that provides a wide spectrum of services. The San Francisco AIDS Foundation, for example, produces and distributes literature, provides counseling, and maintains a hotline in addition to numerous other services. Many of the hotlines are available through the state health departments while others are provided through "AIDS Projects" which are usually staffed with volunteer effort. Some hotlines are merely taped messages which often list another telephone number to call for further information. The hotline from the U.S. Public Health Service is the most widely publicized service, but often is the most difficult to reach. To keep informed of the hotlines that are currently available within each state, contact the respective state health departments.

AID Atlanta of Atlanta, GA	(404) 872-0600
AIDS Action Council of Federated Aids-Related Organizations Washington, DC	(202) 553-2509
AIDS Action Hotline Chicago, IL	(312) 871-5696
AIDS Action Project Howard Brown Memorial Clinic Chicago, IL	(800) 243-2437
AIDS Assistance Network (same as Philadelphia AIDS)	(215) 232-8055
AIDS Center One of Fort Lauderdale, FL (Florida only)	(800) 325-5371
AIDS Council of Northeastern NY	(518) 445-AIDS

AIDS Hotline of AIDS Project of Los Angeles   (213) 871-AIDS
  (10 a.m. - 10 p.m.)   (800) 922-AIDS
  Southern California (toll free)

AIDS Hotline of Indiana   (317) 543-6200

AIDS Hotline of Washington State   (800) 272-2437

AIDS Institute of NY   (800) 462-1884

AIDS Line of Maine   (800) 851-AIDS

AIDS Pastoral Committee   (312) 848-2076
  Chicago, IL

AIDS Project of the East Bay Pacific Center   (415) 420-8181
  for Human Growth (CA)

AIDS Project of Portland, ME   (800) 851-AIDS
  (Mon, Wed evenings, 6 - 9 p.m.; Sat   (207) 774-6877
  morning, 10 a.m. - 1 p.m.)

AIDS Rochester, Inc. (NY)   (716) 232-4430
  (24 hours on call)

ALABAMA AIDS Task Force Hotline   (800) 445-3741
  (1 - 9 p.m.)

Arizona AIDS Information Line   (602) 234-2752
  Phoenix   (602) 234-2753

Arkansas AIDS Hotline   (800) 445-7720

AZT Information Line   (800) 843-9388

Cares Team of Los Angeles   (213) 464-2273

Central New York AIDS Task Force   (315) 475-AIDS

Chicago AIDS Hotline   (800) AID-AIDS

Children and Youth AIDS Hotline   (212) 430-3333
  Albert Einstein College of Medicine, NY
  (9 a.m. - 5 p.m.
  Mon - Fri)

Colorado AIDS Project   (303) 837-0166

Contact   (see local
                                                                  telephone
                                                                  directory)

Dade County Hotline (FL)   (305) 634-4636
   (Callers outside of Dade County)   (800) 443-5046
   (Non-English line for Spanish and Creole)   (305) 324-5148

DC/AIDS Information Line   (202) 332-5295
   (11 a.m. - 10 p.m. Mon - Fri)   (202) 332-AIDS

FARO AIDS Action Council   (415) 553-2509
   Washington, DC

Fenway Community Health Center of Boston   (617) 267-7573

Gay and Lesbian Information and Support   (402) 475-4697
   Lincoln, NE

Gay Men's Health Crisis (NY)   (212) 807-6655

Good Samaritan Project   (816) 561-8780
   Kansas City, MO

Haitian Coalition on AIDS (NY)   (718) 855-0972
   (9 a.m. - 5 p.m. Mon - Fri)

Health Crisis Network (FL)   (305) 634-4636
   (9 a.m. - 9 p.m. Mon - Fri; 10 a.m. - 3 p.m.
   weekends)

Health Education Resource Organization   (301) 945-AIDS
   (HERO) (MD)

Hemophilia Foundation of NY City   (212) 682-5510
   (Hemophilia related information only)

Human Resources Administration AIDS   (212) 645-7070
   Helpline (NY City)

Hyacinth Foundation of New Jersey   (201) 264-8439

Illinois Hotline   (800) AID-AIDS

Kentucky AIDS Information Service   (800) 654-AIDS

Lehigh Valley AIDS Program (PA)   (215) 433-5444
   (24 hours on call)

Long Island Association for AIDS Care, Inc.	(516) 385-AIDS
Mid-Hudson Valley AIDS Task Force (NY) (10 a.m. - 5 p.m. Mon - Fri; 10 a.m. - 9 p.m. Wed)	(914) 993-0607 (914) 993-0606
Minority Task Force on AIDS (NY)	(212) 749-2816
National AIDS Testing Hotline (FL) (9 a.m. - 5 p.m. Mon - Fri)	(800) 356-2437 (305) 748-5900
National Association of People With AIDS (NAPWA)	(415) 553-2509
National Gay Task Force Crisisline (3 p.m. - 9 p.m.)	(800) 221-7044 (212) 807-6016
National Institute on Drug Abuse Rockville, MD	(800) 662-HELP (800) 662-4357
National Sexually Transmitted Diseases Hotline/American Social Health Association	(800) 227-8922
Nebraska AIDS Project Hotline (6 - 11 p.m.)	(800) 782-AIDS
New Jersey AIDS Hotline	(201) 596-0767
New Orleans AIDS Task Force	(504) 522-AIDS (800) 99-AIDS9
New York City AIDS Hotline (9 a.m. - 9 p.m. daily)	(718) 485-8111
New York City Hotline for Health Professionals	(212) 340-4432
New York City Victim Services Agency Hotline	(212) 577-7777
Ohio AIDS Hotline	(800) 332-AIDS
Operation Concern AIDS Worried Well Group of San Francisco	(415) 626-7000
People With AIDS/ARC San Francisco, CA	(415) 861-7309
Philadelphia AIDS Taskforce	(215) 232-8055

Project Inform of San Francisco	(800) 822-7422 (800) 334-7422
PWA (People With Aids) Coalition of New York (10 a.m. - 5 p.m. Mon - Fri)	(212) 242-3900 (212) 627-1810
Rhode Island Project/AIDS Hotline	(401) 277-6502
St. Clare Spellman Center for the Treatment of Persons With AIDS (NY)	(800) 433-AIDS
San Diego AIDS Project Hotline	(619) 260-1304 (619) 543-0300
San Francisco AIDS Activity Project	(415) 863-AIDS
San Francisco AIDS Foundation	(800) FOR-AIDS (415) 864-4376
Sandifer House Hotline (MS)	(800) 826-2961
Southern California AIDS Hotline	(800) 922-AIDS
Southern Tier AIDS Program (NY) (8 a.m. - 5 p.m. Mon - Fri; 7 p.m - 9 p.m. volunteer on beeper)	(607) 723-6520
U.S. Public Health Service (24 hours daily)	(800) 342-AIDS (800) 342-2437
VD National Hotline	(800) 227-8922
Western New York AIDS Program	(716) 847-AIDS
Wisconsin AIDS Hotline	(800) 334-AIDS
Women's AIDS Network (same number as San Francisco AIDS Foundation)	(415) 864-4376 (800) FOR-AIDS

Computerized Sources
of Information

Searching of bibliographic, full-text, and factual databases, along with bulletin boards, represents a primary method for keeping current with the literature and new developments in AIDS research and clinical applications. Included in this section is information concerning online databases, a database on diskette, a CAI program, and bulletin boards.

Almost any database related to the biomedical and social sciences will include some references on AIDS. However, the most efficient approach to online information is to select the database that will provide the highest number of "hits." Highlighted here are some basic files that gave the largest number of postings when searched on BRS or DIALOG, along with some specialized AIDS databases and bulletin boards. Additional information regarding methods and cost of access to the online sources can be obtained from the producers or vendors of the files. The Appendix to this chapter details full information, including addresses and phone number, for database vendors and producers. It must be noted, also, that many of these online databases have print counterparts in the form of indexing or abstracting sources which can be searched manually.

DATABASE SEARCHING

Online searching of databases is available from many vendors worldwide. Three primary vendors will be considered for locating information on AIDS: BRS (including Colleague and BRS AFTERDARK), DIALOG (including Knowledge Index), and MEDLARS, from the National Library of Medicine (NLM). Databases from Wilsonline are briefly mentioned. Additionally, some private sources of databases will be discussed. Sources to consider, but not discussed here include SDC and Mead Data Central's LEXIS/NEXIS system.

Online searching by subject is done with two primary modes of access: subject headings, including controlled vocabulary and descriptors; and free-text searching, usually of the title and abstract. Additional access points to consider when searching many databases are authors and journal titles (for example, several journals now include AIDS in the title).

Since each database has its own method of indexing, and each vendor mounts a database with its own search software, creating variant methods of searching, no attempt has been made to provide an individualized search formulation for each database. Rather, a list of synonyms for AIDS and the HTLV- III virus is provided, leaving the final search formulation to the person needing information. In some cases, however, suggestions are given.

A major caution is given for searching the term "AIDS." In almost every database, searching solely on the word "AIDS" will result in false drops, including "hearing aids," "audiovisual aids," "diagnostic aids," "communication aids," and "aids" used as a verb. If the term "AIDS" is selected for searching, the word should be combined with another word or subject heading, for example, an immunologic concept, the word "virus," or the word "syndrome."

Synonyms or possible terms to consider in searching for AIDS or the HTLV-III virus include:

Disease
> Acquired Immune Deficiency Disease
> Acquired Immunodeficiency Syndrome
> Acquired Immunologic Deficiency Syndrome
> AIDS
> AIDS-Related Complex
> HTLV-III Infection
> HTLV-III-LAV Infection

Virus
> AIDS virus
> ARV
> HIV
> HTLV-III
> Human Immunodeficiency Virus
> Human T-Cell Leukemia Virus Type III
> Human T-Cell Lymphotropic Virus Type III
> Human T-Lymphotropic Virus Type III
> LAV-HTLV-III
> Lymphadenopathy-Associated Virus

ONLINE DATABASES

Listed in this section are databases which provide access to the biomedical literature. For each file, the producer and availability/support services are listed, and where appropriate, coverage, size, update frequency, and print counterpart.

MEDLINE

Producer: National Library of Medicine, 8600 Rockville Pike, Bethesda, MD 20894

Availability: BRS and BRS Colleague (MESH and backfiles); DIALOG (File 154 and backfiles); and NLM

Coverage: 1966 to present (only 1980s literature is relevant)

Size: Over 5,400,000 documents (over 2,150,000, 1980 to present)
Update frequency: Monthly with approx. 25,000 docs.

Print counterpart: *Index Medicus, Index to Dental Literature, International Nursing Index*, plus other selected journals

MEDLINE (MEDLARS On-Line) covers all aspects of biomedicine and health-related sciences. Documents are from the journal literature; approximately 50% contain abstracts online. It remains the database of choice for locating basic biomedical information on both AIDS and the HTLV-III virus. Subject searching on MEDLINE is primarily through *Medical Subject Headings* (*MeSH*), which is a controlled, hierarchical list of subject headings; and additionally by Text Words, which are free-text words in the title and abstract. Relevant *MeSH* terms are:

> ACQUIRED IMMUNODEFICIENCY SYNDROME (beginning 1983)
> AIDS-RELATED COMPLEX (beginning 1987)
> HTLV-III (beginning 1987)

To perform a comprehensive search, especially for literature earlier than the initiation of these subject headings, Text Words must be used.
    The National Library of Medicine produces literature searches on AIDS which are updated quarterly (see Bibliographies/Alerting Services, chapter on Print Sources of Information). The search formulation used for these bibliographies has become more complex over the years as new terminology has developed. The following formulation, taken from Literature Search No. 87-7, is:

SS 1 = ACQUIRED IMMUNODEFICIENCY SYNDROME OR HTLV III OR HUMAN T CELL LEUKEMIA VIRUS AND III (TW) OR AIDS RELATED COMPLEX

SS 2 = (TW) HTLV AND III OR LYMPHADENOPATHY AND ASSOCIATED AND VIRUS OR AIDS AND RELATED AND COMPLEX OR LAV OR HUMAN AND IMMUNODEFICIENCY AND VIRUS OR HIV OR HUMAN AND T AND CELL AND LYMPHOTROPIC AND VIRUS

AND III OR AIDS AND ASSOCIATED AND ALL
RETROVIRUS## OR ARV OR AIDS RES (TA)

SS 3 = 1 OR 2

CANCERLIT

Producer: National Cancer Institute, R.A. Bloch International Cancer
Information Center, 9030 Old Georgetown Road, Bethesda, MD
20892, in cooperation with the National Library of Medicine

Availability: BRS and BRS Colleague (CANR); DIALOG (File 159); and
NLM

Coverage: 1980 to present on BRS; 1963 to present on DIALOG and
MEDLARS (only 1980s literature is relevant)

Size: Over 600,000 documents

Update frequency: Monthly

Print counterpart: None since 1980

    CANCERLIT covers the literature of cancer, including bibliographic
citations and abstracts of journal articles, books, government reports,
meeting abstracts, and dissertations/theses. It is searchable by subject
using Text Words and *Medical Subject Headings* (see *MeSH* in MEDLINE
description above). The high number of postings found in this database is
attributable to the frequency of cancer complications (e.g. Kaposi's
Sarcoma) found in AIDS patients.

EMBASE

Producer: EMBASE, Elsevier Science Publishing Co., Inc., 52 Vanderbilt
Avenue, New York, NY 10017

Availability: BRS and BRS Colleague (EMED); and DIALOG (File 72
and backfiles, 172 and 173)

Coverage: 1980 to present on BRS; 1974 to present on DIALOG (only
1980s literature is relevant)

Size: Over 3 million documents

Update frequency: Every two weeks

Print counterpart: *Excerpta Medica*

EMBASE provides worldwide coverage of the biomedical literature. It includes citations and abstracts to journal articles, conference proceedings, books, and dissertations. While there is a major overlap with MEDLINE, EMBASE is particularly strong in European-based biomedical literature. It is searchable using MALIMET, a highly developed classification scheme, and with free text.

BIOSIS PREVIEWS

Producer: BioSciences Information Service, 2100 Arch Street, Philadelphia, PA 19103

Availability: BRS and BRS Colleague (BIOL and backfile, BIOB; or merged, BIOZ); and DIALOG (Files 5 and 55)

Coverage: 1978 to present on BRS (backfile BIOL is 1970-77); 1969 to present on DIALOG (File 5 is 1969 to present; File 55 is 1981 to present)

Size: Over 5 million records

Update frequency: Monthly on BRS; twice a month on DIALOG

Print counterpart: *Biological Abstracts* and *Biological Abstracts/RRM*

BIOSIS Previews contains bibliographic information and abstracts of books, book chapters, bibliographies, reports, journal literature, meeting papers, and patents in the life sciences. The database is searched using key words, Concept codes, and Biosystematic Codes; the searcher should consult the *BIOSIS Previews Search Guide*. While there is overlap with other databases, especially in coverage of the journal literature, strong points of BIOSIS are its original abstracts and its non-journal coverage.

SCISEARCH

Producer: Institute for Scientific Information, 3501 Market Street, Philadelphia, PA 19104, (215) 386-0100

Availability: DIALOG (File 34, 1984 to present, and File 87, 1981-83; backfiles 94, 1978-80, and 186, 1974-77)

Coverage: 1974 to present (only 1980s literature is relevant)

Size: Over 7 million records (over 3.6 million, 1981 to present)

Update frequency: Bi-weekly with approx. 30,000 items per update

Print counterpart: *Science Citation Index* and *Current Contents*

"SCISEARCH is a multidisciplinary index to the international journal literature of science and technology." Indexed are articles, meeting reports, editorials, letters, etc. Subject searching is via title words. A unique feature is the ability to search by cited reference, so that early, key articles in AIDS research can be traced forward to more current articles which quote a "classic" reference.

COMPREHENSIVE CORE MEDICAL LIBRARY

Producer: BRS Information Technologies, 100 Route 7, Latham, NY 12110

Availability: BRS and BRS Colleague (CCML)

Coverage: 1982 to present

Size: Over 3500 documents

Update frequency: Bi-weekly; concurrent publication with print counterparts

Print counterparts: See *BRS/CCML Database Guide* for a complete list

CCML is a full-text database made available through BRS Information Technologies. Included are the complete texts of major reference works, textbooks and journals in the fields of internal, emergency, and critical care medicine. Clinical information is the primary focus. Subject access is by words in the text. As with any full-text database, searchers should use appropriate methods such as adjacency to narrow their retrieval.

PDQ (PHYSICIAN DATA QUERY)

Producer: National Cancer Institute, R.A. Bloch International Cancer Information Center, 9030 Old Georgetown Road, Bethesda, MD 20892, in cooperation with the National Library of Medicine

Availability: BRS and BRS Colleague (PDQC - PDQ Cancer Information File; PDQD - PDQ Directory File; and PDQP - PDQ Protocol File); and NLM

Coverage: See description below

Size: See description below

Update frequency: Monthly

Print counterpart: None

"PDQ provides physicians with monthly updated information on advances in cancer treatment and it identifies clinical trials for treatment of specific types of cancer." This is a menu-driven database that provides access to:
1. Cancer information file (state-of-the-art treatment information on approx. 85 major cancer types)
2. Directory of physicians file (names, addresses and phone numbers of approx. 10,000 physicians who treat cancer patients)
3. Directory of organizations file (names, addresses and phone numbers of approx. 2,000 organizations and institutions that provide care to cancer patients)
4. Protocol file (summaries of over 1,000 clinical trials for cancer treatment)
PDQ is of special interest to AIDS patients and health care providers because of the potential for complications such as Kaposi's Sarcoma and other forms of cancer.

AMA/NET

Sponsored by the American Medical Association

Producer: SoftSearch, Inc. and American Medical Computing, Ltd., a wholly owned subsidiary of the American Medical Association

Support Services: AMA/NET Customer Support, 1560 Broadway, Suite 900, Denver, CO 80802

AMA/NET, the online medical information network sponsored by the AMA, is intended for the health professional. Access is gained through signing a Network Subscriber Agreement. Included in the network are five online services: literature searches using files such as EMPIRES, MEDLINE through PaperChase, and Social and Economic Aspects of Medicine (SEAM); a diagnostic decision-support tool, DXplain; medical news and public information; computer-based educational programs using MGH-Continuing Medical Education; and electronic mail. Special attention is given to AIDS information in the news and public information section. For example, the Public Information Service includes the CDC's online version of *MMWR, Morbidity & Mortality Weekly Report* on AIDS, and one category of the AP News Service deals specifically with AIDS.

SPECIALIZED DATABASES

The following databases are AIDS-specific, and therefore need not be searched first with the above-mentioned AIDS or HTLV synonyms. Search terms should be geared to the more specialized aspects of the disease, such as Kaposi's Sarcoma, hemophilia, HIV testing, etc. In addition to the online databases, this section contains one program on disk and one computer-assisted program, both for use on an IBM PC.

ACQUIRED IMMUNE DEFICIENCY SYNDROME DATABASE

Producer: Bureau of Hygiene and Tropical Diseases, Keppel Street, London WC1E 7HT, England

Availability: BRS and BRS Colleague (AIDD)

Coverage: 1983 to present

Size: Over 2400 documents

Update frequency: Monthly with approx. 120 docs. per update

Print counterpart: *AIDS and Retroviruses Update*

AIDS is a bibliographic database concentrating on information on "all viruses in the HIV/HTLV family and AIDS-related retroviruses and associated infections." The database includes journal literature and proceedings covering the clinical, research, epidemiological, and public health aspects of the disease. Descriptors use British spellings. Unique features include critically evaluated abstracts, sequencing codes, geographic location, and hardcopy information. Although some bibliographic information overlaps significantly with MEDLINE, there are enough unique references in this database to make it a valuable source.

AIDS EDUCATION FOR THE HEALTH CARE WORKER

Producer: Medi-Sim, Inc., 660 South 4th, P. O. Box 13267, Edwardsville, KS 66113, (913) 441-2881

AIDS Education for the Health Care Worker is a computer-assisted instruction program designed to update the health care professional with factual information about AIDS. Produced in 1987, it covers clinical aspects from diagnosis and treatment to epidemiology, prevention, and risk factors. Included are a self test, bibliography, and resource list. The program is available for use on an IBM PC or compatible.

AIDS KNOWLEDGE BASE

Producer: San Francisco General Hospital, 1001 Potrero Avenue, San Francisco, CA 94110, (Editors: Philip T. Cohen, M.D.; Paul Volberding, M.D.; and Merle Sande, M.D.)

Availability: BRS and BRS Colleague (ASFG)

Update frequency: Twice per week

Print Counterpart: None

The AIDS KNOWLEDGE BASE is an "enhanced online textbook" intended for health care professionals. This full-text file covers all aspects of AIDS, focusing on clinical applications such as treatment, diagnosis, epidemiology (including data from CDC and WHO), HIV testing, pathogenesis, complications, etc. An online Table of Contents feature on Colleague allows easy browsing through the file. As with any full-text file, searchers are cautioned to use appropriate search techniques such as adjacency to eliminate irrelevant retrieval. AIDS KNOWLEDGE BASE promises to be a timely source of information.

BRS COLLEAGUE AIDS LIBRARY

Producer: BRS Information Technologies, 1200 Route 7, Latham, NY 12110

Availability: BRS Colleague

BRS Colleague has created the "AIDS Library," which can be accessed from its main menu. This feature has brought together the following AIDS-related files:

1. AIDS Articles from Colleague's Complete Text Library (AACC). This file is a subset of AIDS-related articles extracted from the vendor's full-text journal collection. Updated twice per week, this file includes the full text of new journal articles on AIDS.

2. MEDLINE References on AIDS (MRAI). For persons who do not wish to search the full MEDLINE database, this is a subset of relevant citations from MEDLINE.

3. AIDS Abstracts from the Bureau of Hygiene and Tropical Diseases (AIDD). This file includes citations and original abstracts from the worldwide AIDS literature (this database is described in more detail above).

4. AIDS KNOWLEDGE BASE. This is a full-text "enhanced online textbook" on AIDS (this database is described in more detail above).

Other databases included in the AIDS Library are PDQ Cancer Information, PDQ Protocols, and Medical and Psychological Previews.
To access the AIDS Library, the user first connects to BRS Colleague through an assigned ID code. At the "COLLEAGUE SERVICES" screen,

enter "1" for the Colleague Medical Search Service, and then "aids" to access the AIDS Library. The following screen will appear to select the appropriate library database:

```
         ACQUIRED IMMUNODEFICIENCY SYNDROME LIBRARY

LIBRARY DATABASES                                      LABEL

AIDS Abstracts from the Bureau of                      AIDD
   Hygiene and Tropical Diseases

AIDS Articles from Colleague's                         AACC
   Complete Text Library

AIDS Knowledge Base from San Francisco                 ASFG
   General Hospital

Medical and Psychological Previews                     PREV

Medline References on AIDS                             MRAI

PDQ Cancer Information                                 PDQC
PDQ Protocols                                          PDQP

ENTER LIBRARY OR DATABASE LABEL
XX--  o
```

CAIN (Computerized AIDS Information Network)

Producer: Gay and Lesbian Community Service Center, Hollywood, CA; and San Francisco AIDS Foundation, 25 Van Ness Street, San Francisco, CA 92138

Availability: Delphi (CAIN, 1213 N. Highland Ave., Hollywood, CA 90038. (213) 464-7400 x277.)

CAIN is a menu-driven system designed for health professionals and persons interested in the educational aspects of AIDS. It includes bibliographic and factual information along with a bulletin board. Menus include Service Providers, Organization Assistance, Research/Clinical Data, Information/Educational Resources, Professional Conferencing, and Electronic Publications.

HIV SEQUENCE DATABASE

Producer: Los Alamos National Laboratory, Los Alamos, NM 87545

This database, produced by the Los Alamos National Laboratory, is funded by the AIDS Program of the National Institute of Allergy and Infectious Diseases. It is available on IBM diskettes and in printed copy, and "will consist of at least four parts: HIV nucleic acid sequences, protein sequences, analyses, and related sequences." This database has been established to track the rapid mutation of the AIDS virus. An initial copy was distributed at the Third International Conference on AIDS, June 1-5, 1987; quarterly updates are anticipated for at least the next three years. Copies are also distributed free of charge to all U.S. medical schools and are available to qualified individuals upon request. For additional information, contact:

> Gerald Myers, Ph.D.
> Theoretical Division
> Group T-10, Mail Stop K710
> Los Alamos National Laboratory
> Los Alamos, NM 87545

OTHER DATABASES

The following list gives some suggestions for other databases to access for AIDS information. It must be emphasized, however, that this list is not intended to be comprehensive. Dependent on the information needed, specialized databases exist for almost every subject area imaginable, many of which will contain some AIDS-related information.

For each database listed below, the vendor(s) is(are) given in parentheses, followed by a brief description of content. The database catalogs and educational materials of the vendor(s) listed in the Appendix to this chapter should be consulted for more detailed information on these and other databases.

ABI/INFORM   (BRS, DIALOG)   AIDS in the workplace from a management viewpoint.

AVLINE (NLM) Audiovisuals.

CATLINE   (NLM)   Monographic, AV, and journal cataloging information.

CINAHL (BRS, DIALOG) Nursing and allied health literature.

FEDERAL RESEARCH IN PROGRESS (DIALOG) Ongoing federally-funded research projects.

GPO MONTHLY CATALOG (BRS, DIALOG) Government documents published by GPO.

HEALTH PLANNING AND ADMINISTRATION (BRS, DIALOG, NLM) Health care administration literature.

MAGAZINE INDEX (BRS, DIALOG) Popular literature.

NATIONAL NEWSPAPER INDEX (BRS, DIALOG) Coverage of major national newspapers.

OCLC EASI Reference (BRS) Monographic, AV, and journal cataloging information.

PHARMACEUTICAL NEWS INDEX (DIALOG) Company and product news from pharmaceutical and health care industries.

PsycINFO (BRS, DIALOG) Psychological literature.

READERS GUIDE' (Wilsonline) Popular literature.

SOCIAL SCIENCE INDEX (Wilsonline) Social sciences literature.

SOCIAL SCISEARCH (BRS, DIALOG) Social sciences literature.

BULLETIN BOARDS/MESSAGING SYSTEMS

Bulletin Boards

AIDS Bulletin Board System
San Francisco, CA
Online phone: (415) 626-1246

CAIN (Computerized AIDS Information Network)
1213 N. Highland Avenue
Hollywood, CA 90038

Accessed through Delphi, (800) 554-4005 (see appendix for information on Delphi; see Specialized Databases, this chapter, for more information on CAIN).

FOG CITY Bulletin Board System
San Francisco, CA
Online phone: (415) 863-9697

Conference Tree Bulletin System - AIDS
San Francisco, CA
Online phone: (415) 626-0258

PhilaMed Bulletin Board System
Philadelphia, PA
Online phone: (215) 848-1152

WAIDS
Human Interaction Research Institute
University of California, Los Angeles
Los Angeles, CA
(213) 479-3028

Messaging Systems

GTE Telemessager AIDS Teleforum Services
GTE TeleMessager Incorporated
910 Royal Lane, Suite 130
Irving, TX 75063
(214) 929-7811

This is a "voice-store-and-forward" messaging service provided to corporations. Messaging commands are: send, receive, reply, direct, and broadcast. A large group of AIDS-associated foundations, action councils, hospitals, public health departments, etc., have joined this network to share information. Access is to members only.

**APPENDIX
VENDORS OF ONLINE INFORMATION**

AMA/NET
AMA/NET Customer Support
1560 Broadway, Suite 900
Denver, CO 80802
(800) 426-2873

BRS Information Technologies
1200 Route 7
Latham, NY 12110
(800) 345-4277
    Access: Telenet, Tymnet
    Over 80 databases, including MEDLINE, AIDS, AIDS KNOWLEDGE BASE, CANCERLIT, and PDQ
    Systems are:
        BRS SEARCH Service -- a command-driven system
        BRS/AFTER DARK -- a command-driven special evening service
        BRS/BRKTHRU -- a menu-driven service

BRS Colleague
BRS Information Technologies
1200 Route 7
Latham, NY 12110
(800) 345-4277
    Access: Telenet, Tymnet
    A biomedical-oriented menu-driven system, providing access to over 80 databases. The AIDS Library, a specialized grouping of AIDS-related databases, is described on pp. 68-9

CAIN
(Computerized AIDS Information Network)
Gay & Lesbian Community Service Center
1213 N. Highland Ave.
Los Angeles, CA 90038
(213) 464-7400 ext. 277

Delphi
3 Blackstone Street
Cambridge, MA 02139
(800) 554-4005
    Provides access for CAIN (Computerized AIDS Information Network)

DIALOG Information Services, Inc.
3460 Hillview Ave.
Palo Alto, CA 94304
(800) 334-2564
    Access: Telenet, Tymnet
    Over 280 databases, including MEDLINE, SCISEARCH, BIOSIS
    Systems are:
        DIALOG -- command-driven service
        Knowledge Index -- menu-driven system

National Library of Medicine
MEDLARS Management Section
8600 Rockville Pike
Bethesda, MD 20209
(800) 638-8480
    Access: Telenet, Tymnet, and direct dial
    Producer (and vendor) of biomedical databases, including MEDLINE,
    CANCERLIT, and PDQ

Wilsonline
H.W. Wilson Company
950 University Avenue
Bronx, NY 10452
(800) 367-6770
(800) 462-6060 (New York State)

Print Sources
of Information

The information contained in this chapter is intended to provide access points primarily to the professional health sciences literature, where major developments in AIDS research are reported. Because the literature on AIDS is expanding so rapidly, only selected core journal articles and books are listed. Rather, the focus is on access points for finding up-to-date information, such as bibliographies, specialized AIDS journals, and biomedical journals that routinely contains AIDS-related materials.

Sections included below are: Indexing/Abstracting Journals; Bibliographies/Alerting Services; Selected Scientific Journal Articles; Specialized Journals/Newsletters; and Reference Sources/Monographs.

INDEXING/ABSTRACTING JOURNALS

Major sources for accessing the literature are indexing, and abstracting journals. Since the online versions of these sources are more current, they are mentioned within the chapter, Computerized Sources of Information, in the annotation, "Print Counterpart." For example, *Index Medicus* is a major source to check for current journal literature; however, it is mentioned under MEDLINE. Other indexing/abstracting journals mentioned in Computerized Sources of Information include *Biological Abstracts* (see BIOSIS); *Science Citation Index* (see SCISEARCH); and *Excerpta Medica* (see EMBASE).

BIBLIOGRAPHIES/ALERTING SERVICES

Alerting services (current awareness services or selective dissemination of information) generate updates of current literature. With the exception of SDILINE, the services listed here are geared specifically to the AIDS literature.

The bibliographies listed here are compilations of references on AIDS-related literature. It must be remembered that these lists will be quickly outdated. However, they are still useful in looking at the retrospective literature.

Alerting Services

AIDS.
Oncology Information Service, Medical and Dental Library, University of Leeds, Leeds LS2 9JT, United Kingdom.

A monthly current literature scanning service that includes between 150 and 200 international items per month, from over 1300 biomedical journals. Abstracts/annotations are provided.

AIDS Literature & News Review.
ISSN 0893-8633
University Publishing Group, 107 East Church Street, Frederick, MD 21701. (800) 654-8188

A monthly alerting service that provides bibliographic citations and summaries of literature on AIDS. Professional journals and reports are scanned, along with articles from major newspapers and law journals.

ASCATOPICS - AIDS - IMMUNE DEFICIENCY STATES (S0713).
Weekly computer-generated bibliography.
Institute for Scientific Information, 3501 Market Street, Philadelphia, PA 19104. (215) 386-0100 and (800) 523- 1850, ext. 1585.

SDILINE.
A monthly update of the MEDLINE database (see MEDLINE, Computerized Sources of Information). The user determines his own profile for the update.

Bibliographies

National Library of Medicine Literature Search No. 83-1. **Acquired Immunodeficiency Syndrome (AIDS).** January 1980 through April 1983. *(179 citations, including Addendum).*

National Library of Medicine Literature Search No. 83-5. **Acquired Immunodeficiency Syndrome (AIDS). Update and Supplement.** May 1983 through August 1983. *(215 citations, including Addendum).*

National Library of Medicine Literature Search No. 83-25. **Acquired Immunodeficiency Syndrome (AIDS): Second Quarterly Update and**

Supplement. September 1983 through December 1983. *(344 citations, including Addendum).*

National Library of Medicine Literature Search No. 84-9. **Acquired Immunodeficiency Syndrome (AIDS): Third Quarterly Update and Supplement.** January 1984 through April 1984. *(387 citations, including Addendum).*

National Library of Medicine Literature Search No. 84-18. **Acquired Immunodeficiency Syndrome (AIDS): Fourth Quarterly Update and Supplement.** May 1984 through July 1984. *(406 citations, including Addendum).*

National Library of Medicine Literature Search No. 84-32. **Acquired Immunodeficiency Syndrome (AIDS): Fifth Update and Supplement.** August 1984 through December 1984. *(646 citations, including Addendum).*

National Library of Medicine Literature Search No. 84-33. **Human T-Cell Leukemia/Lymphoma Virus (HTLV).** January 1982 through September 1984. *(234 citations).*

National Library of Medicine Literature Search No. 85-4. **Acquired Immunodeficiency Syndrome (AIDS): Sixth Update.** January 1985 through April 1985. *(582 citations, including Addendum).*

National Library of Medicine Literature Search No. 85-8. **Childhood Immunodeficiency Disorders.** January 1983 through April 1985. *(343 citations in English).*

National Library of Medicine Literature Search No. 85-16. **Acquired Immunodeficiency Syndrome (AIDS): Seventh Update and Supplement.** May 1985 through August 1985. *(747 citations, including Addendum).*

National Library of Medicine Literature Search No. 85-20. **Acquired Immunodeficiency Syndrome (AIDS): Eighth Update.** September 1985 through December 1985. *(577 citations).*

National Library of Medicine Literature Search No. 86-3. **Acquired Immunodeficiency Syndrome (AIDS): Ninth Update.** January 1986 through March 1986. *(478 citations).*

National Library of Medicine Literature Search No. 86-6. **HTLV-III Antibody Testing: Efficiency and Impact on Public Health.** January 1984 through June 1986. *(420 citations in English).*

National Library of Medicine Literature Search No. 86-9. **Acquired Immunodeficiency Syndrome (AIDS): Tenth Update.** April 1986 through June 1986. *(552 citations).*

National Library of Medicine Literature Search No. 86-13. **Acquired Immunodeficiency Syndrome (AIDS): Eleventh Update.** July 1986 through September 1986. *(680 citations).*

National Library of Medicine Literature Search No. 86-16. **Acquired Immunodeficiency Syndrome (AIDS): Twelfth Update.** October 1986 through December 1986. *(676 citations, including Addendum).*

National Library of Medicine Literature Search No. 87-3. **Acquired Immunodeficiency Syndrome (AIDS): Thirteenth Update.** January 1987 through March 1987. *(684 citations).*

National Library of Medicine Literature Search No. 87-7. **Acquired Immunodeficiency Syndrome (AIDS): Fourteenth Update.** April 1987 through June 1987. *(890 citations).*

National Library of Medicine Literature Search No. 87-13. **Acquired Immunodeficiency Syndrome (AIDS): Fifteenth Update.** July 1987 through September 1987. *(845 citations).*

**(Beginning in 1988, a subscription service to the quarterly NLM AIDS Literature Searches is available as AIDS Bibliography, GPO List ID: AID88; the annual subscription is $12. To obtain single copies of the National Library of Medicine Literature Searches listed above, send a self-addressed gummed label along with LS numbers and titles to: Literature Search Program, Reference Section, National Library of Medicine, Bethesda, MD 20894. Older Literature Searches may no longer be available, but can be found at most medical school libraries.)

National Library of Medicine. Reference Section. **AIDS Bibliography, 1986-1987.** Available from National Technical Information Service, Springfield, VA 22161. Order no. PB87-190716/GBB. ($24.95 plus $3 handling). Cumulates the Literature Searches for January 1986 through April 1987. 2700 citations.

Tyckoson, David A., ed. **AIDS 1987.** Phoenix, AZ: Oryx Press, 1987. 160 p. ISBN 0-89774-434-9.

Tyckoson, David A., ed. **AIDS 1986.** Phoenix, AZ: Oryx Press, 1986. 96 p. ISBN 0-89774-323-7. (also advertised as *AIDS (Acquired Immune Deficiency Syndrome)*, 2nd ed., vol. 7 of Oryx Science Bibliographies).

Tyckoson, David A., ed. **AIDS: Acquired Immune Deficiency Syndrome.** Phoenix, AZ: Oryx Press, 1985. 64 p. ISBN 0-89774-203-6. (Also advertised as *AIDS (Acquired Immune Deficiency Syndrome)*, vol. 1 of Oryx Science Bibliographies).

SELECTED SCIENTIFIC JOURNAL ARTICLES

The following list of journal articles has been selected from the biomedical literature. The emphasis is primarily clinical, and an attempt has been made to cover most aspects of the disease. These articles will be available in most health sciences libraries, and many have extensive bibliographies. Inclusion here is not necessarily an endorsement of the article; many excellent articles were not included.

The journals which contain these articles also represent a core list of biomedical journals that routinely publish papers on AIDS, and could be regularly scanned to keep up-to-date. This list includes: *Annals of Internal Medicine; JAMA, Journal of the American Medical Association; MMWR, Morbidity and Mortality Weekly Report; New England Journal of Medicine,* and *Science.*

American Academy of Pediatrics. "School Attendance of Children and Adolescents with Human T Lymphotropic Virus III/ Lymphadenopathy-Associated Virus Infection." **Pediatrics** 77(March 1986):430-2.

Ammann, Arthur J. "The Acquired Immunodeficiency Syndrome in Infants and Children." **Annals of Internal Medicine** 103(November 1985):734-7.

Barbour, Stephen David. "Acquired Immunodeficiency Syndrome of Childhood." **Pediatric Clinics of North America** 34(February 1987):247-68.

Barre-Sinoussi, Francoise; Chermann, J.C.; Rey, F., et al. "Isolation of a T-Lymphotropic Retrovirus from a Patient at Risk for Acquired Immune Deficiency Syndrome (AIDS)." **Science** 220(May 20, 1983):868-71.

Barre-Sinoussi, Francoise; Mathur-Wagh, Usha; Rey, Francoise, et al. "Isolation of Lymphadenopathy-Associated Virus (LAV) and Detection of LAV Antibodies from US Patients with AIDS." **JAMA** 253(March 22/29, 1985):1737-9.

Bayer, Ronald; Fox, Daniel M.; and Willis, David P. "AIDS: The Public Context of an Epidemic." **Milbank Quarterly** 64(Supplement 1, 1986):1-182. (A collection of 8 articles.)

Board of Trustees Report. "Prevention and Control of Acquired Immunodeficiency Syndrome; An Interim Report." **JAMA** 258(October 16, 1987):2097-2103.

"Classification System for Human T-Lymphotropic Virus Type III/Lymphadenopathy-Associated Virus Infections." **MMWR** 35(May 23, 1986):334-9.

"Coolfont Report: A PHS Plan for Prevention and Control of AIDS and the AIDS Virus." **Public Health Reports** 101(July-August 1986):341-8.

Cooney, Thomas G., and Ward, Thomas T. "AIDS and Other Medical Problems in the Male Homosexual." **Medical Clinics of North America** 70(May 1986):497-725. (A collection of 12 articles, of which 6 are on AIDS.)

Curran, James W. "The Epidemiology and Prevention of the Acquired Immunodeficiency Syndrome." **Annals of Internal Medicine** 103(November 1985):657-62.

Curran, James W.; Morgan, W. Meade; Hardy, Ann M., et al. "The Epidemiology of AIDS: Current Status and Future Prospects." **Science** 229(September 27, 1985):1352-7.

Fauci, Anthony S. "Current Issues in Developing a Strategy for Dealing with the Acquired Immunodeficiency Syndrome." **Proceedings of the National Academy of Sciences** 83(December 1986):9278-83.

Fauci, Anthony S.; Masur, Henry; Gelmann, Edward P., et al. "The Acquired Immunodeficiency Syndrome: An Update." **Annals of Internal Medicine** 102(June 1985):800-13.

Francis, Donald P.; Jaffe, Harold W.; Fultz, Patricia N., et al. "The Natural History of Infection With Lymphadenopathy-Associated Virus Human T-Lymphotropic Virus Type III." **Annals of Internal Medicine** 103(November 1985):719-22.

Francis, Donald P., and Petricciani, John C. "The Prospects for and Pathways Toward a Vaccine for AIDS." **New England Journal of Medicine** 313(December 19, 1985):1586-90.

Friedland, Gerald H., and Klein, Robert S. "Transmission of the Human Immunodeficiency Virus." **New England Journal of Medicine** 317(October 29, 1987):1125-1135.

Gallo, Robert C. "The AIDS Virus." **Scientific American** 256(January 1987):47-56. (Part 1 of this two-part article was: "The First Human Retrovirus." *Scientific American* 255:88-98, December 1986.)

Gallo, Robert C.; Salahuddin, Syed Z.; Popovic, Mikulas, et al. "Frequent Detection and Isolation of Cytopathic Retroviruses (HTLV-III) from Patients with AIDS and at Risk for AIDS." **Science** 224(May 4, 1983):500-3.

Gallo, Robert C., and Wong-Staal, Flossie. "A Human T- Lymphotropic Retrovirus (HTLV-III) as the Cause of the Acquired Immunodeficiency Syndrome." **Annals of Internal Medicine** 103(November 1985):679-89.

Gerberding, J. Louise, and the University of California, San Francisco Task Force on AIDS. "Recommended Infection-Control Policies for

Patients With Human Immunodeficiency Virus Infection: An Update." **New England Journal of Medicine** 315(December 11, 1986):1562-4.

Gostin, Larry, and Curran, William J. "AIDS Screening, Confidentiality, and the Duty to Warn." **American Journal of Public Health** 77(March 1987):361-5.

Gostin, Larry, and Curran, William J. "Legal Control Measures for AIDS: Reporting Requirements, Surveillance, Quarantine, and Regulation of Public Meeting Places." **American Journal of Public Health** 77(February 1987):214-8.

Guinan, Mary E., and Hardy, Ann. "Epidemiology of AIDS in Women in the United States: 1981 Through 1986." **JAMA** 257(April 17, 1987):2039-42.

Handsfield, H. Hunter; Cummings, M. Jeanne; and Swenson, Paul D. "Prevalence of Antibody to Human Immunodeficiency Virus and Hepatitus B Surface Antigen in Blood Samples Submitted to a Hospital Laboratory; Implications for Handling Specimens." **JAMA** 258(December 18, 1987):3395-7.

Hardy, Ann M.; Allen, James R.; Morgan, W. Meade, et al. "The Incidence Rate of Acquired Immunodeficiency Syndrome in Selected Populations." **JAMA** 253(January 11, 1985):215-20.

Hilgartner, Margaret W. "AIDS in the Transfused Patient." **American Journal of Diseases of Children** 141(February 1987):194-8.

"International Conference on Acquired Immunodeficiency Syndrome." **Annals of Internal Medicine** 103(November 1985):653-781. (A collection of 25 papers; some are listed separately in this bibliography.)

Jaffe, Harold W.; Bregman, Dennis J.; and Selik, Richard M. "Acquired Immune Deficiency Syndrome in the United States: The First 1,000 Cases." **Journal of Infectious Diseases** 148(August 1983):339-45.

Kaminsky, L.S.; McHugh, T.; Stites, D., et al. "High Prevalence of Antibodies to Acquired Immune Deficiency Syndrome (AIDS)-Associated Retrovirus (ARV) in AIDS and Related Conditions but not in Other Disease States." **Proceedings of the National Academy of Sciences USA** 82(1985):5535-5539.

Kaplan, Lawrence D.; Wofsy, Constance B.; and Volberding, Paul A. "Treatment of Patients With Acquired Immunodeficiency Syndrome and Associated Manifestations." **JAMA** 257(March 13, 1987):1367-74.

Koop, C. Everett. "Surgeon General's Report on Acquired Immune Deficiency Syndrome." **JAMA** 256(November 28, 1986):2783-9.

Landesman, Sheldon; Minkoff, Howard; Holman, Susan, et al. "Serosurvey of Human Immunodeficiency Virus Infection in Parturients; Implications for Human Immunodeficiency Virus Testing Programs of Pregnant Women." **JAMA** 258(November 20, 1987):2701-3.

Lang, William; Anderson, Robert E.; Perkins, Herbert, et al. "Clinical, Immunologic, and Serologic Findings in Men at Risk for Acquired Immunodeficiency Syndrome: The San Francisco Men's Health Study." **JAMA** 257(January 16, 1987):326-30.

Levy, Jay A.; Hoffman, Anthony D.; Kramer, Susan M., et al. "Isolation of Lymphocytopathic Retroviruses from San Francisco Patients with AIDS." **Science** 225(August 24, 1984):840-842.

Levy, Jay A.; Kaminsky, Lawrence S.; Morrow, W.J.W., et al. "Infection by the Retrovirus Associated with the Acquired Immunodeficiency Syndrome: Clinical, Biological and Molecular Features." **Annals of Internal Medicine** 103(November 1985):694-9.

Lewis, Hilary E. "Acquired Immunodeficiency Syndrome; State Legislative Activity." **JAMA** 258(November 6, 1987):2410-4.

McCray, Eugene. "Occupational Risk of the Acquired Immunodeficiency Syndrome Among Health Care Workers." **New England Journal of Medicine** 314(April 24, 1986):1127-32.

Matthews, Gene W., and Neslund, Verla S. "The Initial Impact of AIDS on Public Health Law in the United States -- 1986." **JAMA** 257(January 16, 1987):344-52.

Melbye, Mads. "The Natural History of Human T-Lymphotropic Virus-III Infection: The Cause of AIDS." **British Medical Journal** 292(January 4, 1986):5-12.

Minkoff, Howard L. "Care of Pregnant Women Infected With Human Immunodeficiency Virus." **JAMA** 258(November 20, 1987):2714-7.

Morgan, W. Meade, and Curran, James W. "Acquired Immunodeficiency Syndrome: Current and Future Trends." **Public Health Reports** 101 (September-October 1986):459-65.

Murray, Henry W.; Hillman, Janice K.; Rubin, Berish Y., et al. "Patients at Risk for AIDS-Related Opportunistic Infection." **New England Journal of Medicine** 313(December 12, 1985):1504-10.

Osterholm, Michael T.; Bowman, Robert J.; Chopek, Michael W., et al. "Screening Donated Blood and Plasma for HTLV-III Antibody: Facing More Than One Crisis." **New England Journal of Medicine** 312(May 2, 1985):1185-9.

Peterman, Thomas A., and Curran, James W. "Sexual Transmission of Human Immunodeficiency Virus." **JAMA** 256(October 24/31, 1986):2222-6.

Peterman, Thomas A.; Jaffe, Harold W.; Feorino, Paul M., et al. "Transfusion-Associated Acquired Immunodeficiency Syndrome in the United States." **JAMA** 254(November 22/29, 1985):2913-7.

PHS Executive Task Force on AIDS. "Public Health Service Plan for the Prevention and Control of Acquired Immune Deficiency Syndrome (AIDS)." **Public Health Reports** 100(September-October 1985):453-5.

Popovic, M.; Sarngadharan, M.G.; Reed, E., et al. "Detection, Isolation, and Continuous Production of Cytopathic Retroviruses (HTLV-III) from Patients with AIDS and Pre-AIDS." **Science** 224(May 4, 1984):497-500.

"Public Health Service Guidelines for Counseling and Antibody Testing to Prevent HIV Infection and AIDS." **MMWR** 36(August 14, 1987):509-15.

"Recommendations for Preventing Transmission of Infection with Human T-Lymphotropic Virus Type III/Lymphadenopathy-Associated Virus in the Workplace." **MMWR** 34(November 15, 1985):682-94.

"Recommendations for Prevention of HIV Transmission in Health-Care Settings." **MMWR** 36(Suppl. no. 2S, August 21, 1987):1S-18S.

"Revision of the Case Definition of Acquired Immunodeficiency Syndrome for National Reporting -- United States." **MMWR** 34(June 28, 1985):373-5.

"Revision of the CDC Surveillance Case Definition for Acquired Immunodeficiency Syndrome." **MMWR** 36(Suppl. no. 1S, August 14, 1987):1S-15S.

Sarngadharan, M.G.; Popovic, M.; Bruch, L., et al. "Antibodies Reactive with Human T-Lymphotropic Retroviruses (HTLV-III) in the Serum of Patients With AIDS." **Science** 224(May 4, 1984):506-8.

Schupbach, Jorg; Gilden, Raymond V.; Gonda, Matthew A., et al. "Serological Analysis of a Subgroup of Human T-Lymphotropic Retroviruses (HTLV-III) Associated with AIDS." **Science** 224(May 4, 1984):503-5.

Siegel, Karolyn, guest editor. "AIDS Education: The Public Health Challenge." **Health Education Quarterly** 13(Winter 1986):285-422. (Issue contains 10 health education articles.)

"Update: Acquired Immunodeficiency Syndrome -- United States." **MMWR** 35(December 12, 1986):757-60, 765-6.

"Update: Human Immunodeficiency Virus Infections in Health Care Workers Exposed to Blood of Infected Patients." **MMWR** 36(May 22, 1987):285-9.

Winkelstein, Warren; Lyman, David M.; Padian, Nancy, et al. "Sexual Practices and Risk of Infection by the Human Immunodeficiency Virus: The San Francisco Men's Health Study." **JAMA** 257(January 16, 1987):321-5.

SPECIALIZED JOURNALS/NEWSLETTERS

The following journals or newsletters are directed specifically at publishing AIDS information. Some are international scientific journals, while others are national newsletters. A few local newsletters are included as examples of the types of materials that are available at that level.

AIDS *see* **AIDS-Berichte.**

AIDS (Seattle, WA).
  Quarterly.
  Prevention Project, Seattle, WA

AIDS: An International Bimonthly Journal.
  Vol. 1- , May 1987- .
  Vol. 1, 1987 to consist of 4 issues; bi-monthly beginning with V.2, 1988.
  ISSN 0269-9370
  Gower Academic Journals, 34 Cleveland Street, London W1P 5FB, United Kingdom.

  Publishes papers of original research related to AIDS.

AIDS Action Update.
  Newsletter.
  FARO AIDS Action Council, 111 S. 1/2 Independence Ave. SE, Washington, DC 20003. (202) 547-3101

AIDS Alert.
  Vol. 1- , January 1986- .
  Monthly.
  ISSN 0887-0292
  American Health Consultants, Inc., 67 Peachtree Park Dr., N.E. #220, Atlanta, GA 30309. (404) 351-4523

AIDS & Public Policy.
Vol. 1- , July 1986- .
Bi-monthly.
ISSN 0887-3852
University Publishing Group, Inc., 107 E. Church St., Frederick, MD 21701.

AIDS-Berichte.
Vol. 1- , 1985- .
Grosse Verlag, Berlin, West Germany.

German language.

AIDS-Forschung.
Vol. 1- , January 1986- .
ISSN 0179-3098
Verlag R.S. Schulz, Berger Strasse 8 Bis 10,8136 Percha Am Starnberger See, West Germany.

German language.

AIDS Information Exchange.
Vol. 1- , June 1984- .
Irregular.
ISSN 0891-7426
United States Conference of Mayors, 1620 Eye Street NW, Washington, DC 20006.

AIDS Law & Litigation Reporter *see* section on Reference Sources/Monographs, this chapter, for details.

AIDS Literature & News Review *see* Bibliographies/Alerting Services, this chapter, for details (ISSN 0893-8633).

AIDS Medical Update.
10-12 issues per year.
Center for Interdisciplinary Research in Immunology and Diseases at UCLA, 12-248 Factor Building, Department of Microbiology and Immunology, UCLA School of Medicine, Los Angeles, CA 90024. (213) 825-1510

AIDS Newsletter.
Vol. 1- , 1985- .
Monthly newsletter.
Massachusetts Department of Public Health/Boston Department of Health and Hospitals.
Boston Department of Health and Hospitals, House Officers Building, Room 321, 818 Harrison Avenue, Boston, MA 02118. (617) 424-4748

AIDS Newsletter.
Vol. 1- , 1986- .
ISSN 0268-8360
Bureau of Hygiene and Tropical Diseases, Keppel Street, London WC1E 7HT England.

AIDS Patient Care; A Magazine for Health Professionals.
Vol. 1- , June 1987- .
3 issues in 1987; bi-monthly thereafter.
ISSN 0893-5068
Mary Ann Liebert, Inc., 1651 Third Avenue, New York, NY 10128. (212) 289-2300 or (800) 526-5368

AIDS Policy & Law.
v. 1- , January 29, 1986- .
Bi-weekly.
ISSN 0887-1493
BURAFF Publications, Inc., 2445 M Street, N.W., Suite 275, Washington, DC 20037. (202) 452-7889.

The bi-weekly newsletter on legislation, regulation, and litigation concerning AIDS.

AIDS Record.
Vol. 1- , December 1, 1986- .
Semi-monthly.
ISSN 0891-3765
BIO-DATA Publishers, 1518 K Street NW-Mezzanine, Washington, DC 20005.

Subscription includes a telephone resource service and *The AIDS Record Directory.*

AIDS Report.
Vol. 1- , August 1987- .
Monthly newsletter.
FNP Health Division, 155 Post Road East, PO Box 71, Westport, CT 06881. (203) 227-6596 or (203) 227-8779

AIDS Research.
Vol. 1-2, 1983-1986.
6 issues in vol. 1; 4 issues in vol. 2; supplement to vol. 2.
ISSN 0737-6006
Continued by *AIDS Research and Human Retroviruses*.

AIDS Research and Human Retroviruses.
Vol. 3- , 1987- .
Quarterly with supplement. Continues *AIDS Research*.
ISSN 0889-2229
Mary Ann Liebert, Inc., 1651 Third Avenue, New York, NY 10128.

Includes peer-reviewed original articles on basic research and clinical observations of AIDS. Also covers studies pertaining to cancer, degenerative diseases and the immune system.

Aids Surveillance Monthly Update.
October 1986- .
Bureau of Communicable Disease Control, New York State Department of Public Health, Albany, NY 12237.

AIDS Treatment News.
Bi-weekly.
John S. James, P. O. Box 411256, San Francisco, CA 94141.

Collects information on experimental and alternative treatments. Also examines the ethical and public issues related to AIDS treatment research.

AIDS Update.
Monthly.
Lambda Legal Defense and Education Fund, 666 Broadway, New York, NY 10012.

AIDS Update.
Vol. 1- , 1986- .
Michigan Department of Public Health, Lansing, MI

AIDS Weekly Surveillance Report.
Weekly.

CDC, AIDS Surveillance Section, P.O. Box 5528, Building 3, Room 5B-1, 1600 Clifton Road, Atlanta, GA 30307-0528. (404) 639-3472

Includes CDC statistical data. Free.

ECLIPSE; The Shanti Project Newsletter.
Shanti Project, 525 Howard Street, San Francisco, CA 94105. (415) 777-CARE

Healing AIDS.
Monthly newsletter.
3835 20th Street, San Francisco, CA 94114. (415) 864- 6870

Network News; A Semi-Monthly Publication of the National AIDS Network.
Vol. 1- , 1987- .
Semi-monthly.
National AIDS Network, 1012 14th Street NW, Suite 601, Washington, DC 20005.

Official Newsletter of the National Coalition of Gay STD Services *see Sexual Health Reports*

PWA Coalition Newsline.
Monthly newsletter.
People with AIDS Coalition, 263A West 19th Street, Room 125, New York, NY 10011. (212) 627-1810

Sexual Health Reports.
Vol. 9, No. 1- , Fall 1987- .
Quarterly.
National Coalition of Gay STD Services, P.O. Box 239, Milwaukee, WI 53201. (414) 277-7671

Includes reprints from *MMWR.*

REFERENCE SOURCES/MONOGRAPHS

The following reference sourses/monographs were selected to give an overall view of AIDS. They are clinically-oriented and many deal with the social/psychological aspects of the disease. With a few exceptions, the references are from the professional literature. Inclusion here should not be considered an endorsement of the material; other excellent books are available but were not selected.

AIDS: Epidemiological and Clinical Studies. Waltham, MA: Massachusetts Medical Society, 1987. 349 p. ISBN 0-910133-19-0.

Reprints from the *New England Journal of Medicine*, 1981-1987.

AIDS: The Safety of Blood and Blood Products, edited by J.C. Petricciani, et al. Chichester, NY: Published on behalf of the World Health Organization by Wiley, 1987. 374 p. 0-471913383.

AIDS Law & Litigation Reporter. Frederick, MD: University Publishing Group, 1986- . Annual. ISBN 1-55572-003-X.

In addition to full-text coverage of federal, state and local court cases, surveys of proposed and enacted legislation and statutes, and analysis of current thinking regarding AIDS law and litigation, the *Reporter* features a monthly newsletter.

AIDS Project Los Angeles. **AIDS: A Self-Care Manual.** Los Angeles, CA: IBS Press, 1987. 306 p. 0-9616605-1-1 (pbk.).

300 pages of resource material related to medical, psychosocial, and pratical aspects of AIDS.

AIDS Reference & Research Collections: 1980-1988. Frederick, MD: University Publishing Group, 1988.

Complete Two-Volume Set. ISBN 1-55572-002-1.
History of AIDS. ISBN 1-55572-004-8.
AIDS Literature. ISBN 1-55572-005-6.
Hearings & Special Reports. ISBN 1-55572-006-4.
AIDS-Related Services. ISBN 1-55572-007-2.

AIDS, The Workplace Issues. New York: AMA Membership Publications Division, American Management Association, 1985. 81 p. ISBN 0-8144-2321-3.

Altman, Dennis. **AIDS in the Mind of America.** New York: Anchor Press/Doubleday, 1987. 228 p. ISBN 0-385-19523-0.

Written by a political scientist about the politics of AIDS in the United States.

American Foundation for AIDS Research, comp. **AmFAR Directory of Experimental Treatments for AIDS and ARC. Vol. 1.** New York: Mary Ann Liebert, Inc., June 1987. ISBN 0-913113-11- 8; ISSN 0893-9942.

> Updated with bi-monthly supplements. This work is arranged alphabetically by experimental drug and includes information on physician investigators and current research, experimental treatment centers, and a bibliography of treatment review articles. It has an Index to Physician Investigators.

Baumgartner, Gail Henderson. **AIDS, Psychosocial Factors in the Acquired Immune Deficiency Syndrome.** Springfield, IL: Thomas, 1985. 113 p. ISBN 0-398-05188-7.

Blanchet, Kevin D., ed. **AIDS, A Health Care Management Response.** Rockville, MD: Aspen Publishers, 1988. ISBN 0-87189-877-2.

Broder, Samuel. **AIDS: Modern Concepts and Therapeutic Challenges.** New York: Marcel Dekker, Inc., 1987. 369 p. ISBN 0-8247-7649-6.

> Emphasis on medical aspects of AIDS with over 1000 references.

Center for Interdisciplinary Research in Immunology and Disease at UCLA. **AIDS Reference Guide for Medical Professionals.** 2nd ed. Los Angeles, CA: CIRID, 1986. Annual.

> Published in loose-leaf format, this work overviews AIDS, the CDC definitions, experimental therapies, and lists national resources.

Cole, Helene M., and Lundberg, George D. **AIDS, From the Beginning.** Chicago, IL: American Medical Association, 1986. 441 p. ISBN 0-89970-207-4 (pbk.).

> A collection of reprints of the articles and news items, many originally published in *JAMA, Journal of the American Medical Association.*

Curran, William J.; Gosten, Larry O.; Clark, Mary. **Acquired Immunodeficiency Syndrome: Legal and Regulatory Policy.** Washington, DC: Department of Health and Human Services, 1986.

Reprint. Originally published: Boston, MA: Harvard University School of Public Health, Department of Health Policy and Management, 1986.

Dalton, Harlon L.; Burns, Scott; and the Yale AIDS Law Project. **AIDS and the Law: A Guide for the Public.** New Haven, CT: Yale University Press, 1987. 382 p. ISBN 0-300-04077-6; ISBN 0-300-04078-4 (pbk.).

Daniels, Victor G. **AIDS, The Acquired Immune Deficiency Syndrome.** 2nd ed. Lancaster; Boston: MTP Press, 1987. 155 p. ISBN 0-7462-0035-8.

Delaney, Martin, and Goldblum, Peter. **Strategies for Survival: A Gay Men's Health Manual for the Age of AIDS.** New York: St. Martin's Press, Inc., 1987. ISBN 0-312-00558-X (pbk.).

Discusses the establishment of a personal health plan and addresses such issues as sexual practices, substance abuse, exercise and nutrition, and stress.

DeVita, Vincent, et al., eds. **AIDS: Etiology, Diagnosis, Treatment, and Prevention.** Philadelphia: Lippincott, 1985. 352 p. ISBN 0-397-50697-X.

Feldman, Douglas A., and Johnson, Thomas M., eds. **The Social Dimensions of AIDS: Method and Theory.** New York: Praeger Publishers, 1986. 274 p. ISBN 0-275-92110-7.

Provides an overview of AIDS from a social viewpoint including the aspects of anthropology, edidemiology, and sociology.

Frumkin, Lyn Robert, and Leonard, John Martin. **Questions and Answers on AIDS: The Biomedical and Social Impact of the Acquired Immunodeficiency Syndrome.** Oradell, NJ: Medical Economics Books, 1987. 190 p. ISBN 0-87489-461-1.

Greenly, Mike. **Chronicle: The Human Side of AIDS.** New York: Irvington Publishers, Inc., 1986. 422 p. ISBN 0-8290-1800-X.

Hyde, Margaret O., and Forsyth, Elizabeth H. **AIDS: What Does It Mean to You?** New York: Walker and Company, 1987. ISBN 0-8027-6706-0; ISBN 0-8027-6705-2 (lib. ed.).

Keeling, Richard P., ed. **AIDS on the College Campus.** Rockville, MD: American College Health Association, 1986. (ACHA Special Report.)

> Discusses administrative issues and policies, confidentiality, HTLV-III antibody testing, housing policies, educational resources and risk assessment.

Klein, Eva, ed. **Acquired Immunodeficiency Syndrome.** Basel: Karger, 1986. 398 p. ISBN 3-8055-4156-2. (*Progress in Allergy*, Vol. 37.)

Kubler-Ross, Elisabeth. **AIDS: The Ultimate Challenge.** New York: Macmillan, to be published in January 1988. 320 p. ISBN 0-02-567170-7.

> Writen by a leading authority on death and dying, the author speaks to those affected by AIDS as well as those who fear the disease.

Kulstad, Ruth., ed. **AIDS: Papers From <u>SCIENCE</u>, 1982-1985.** Washington, DC: American Association for the Advancement of Science, 1986. 653 p. ISBN 0-87168-313-X; ISBN 0-87168-281-8 (pbk.).

> A chronological arrangement of 108 research papers and news reports from the journal *Science* between August 1982 and September 1985.

Lesbian and Gay Rights Project. **AIDS: Basic Documents and Model Statutes.** New York: The Project, 1987.

> A free publication that includes model laws concerning testing and anti-discrimination. Contact Nan D. Hunter, Lesbian and Gay Rights Project, ACLU, 132 W. 43rd Street, New York, NY 10036.

Malinowski, H. Robert, and Perry, Gerald J. **The AIDS Information Sourcebook.** Phoenix, AZ: Oryx Press, 1987. 112 p. ISBN 0-89774-419-5.

> A guide to sources of information for persons seeking "professional advice, counseling, testing, and treatment.

Martelli, Leonard J.; with Peltz, Fran D., and Messina, William. **When Someone You Know Has AIDS: A Practical Guide.** New York: Crown Publishers, Inc., 1987. 240 p. ISBN 0-517-56555-2; ISBN 0-517-56556-0 (pbk.).

> Includes testimonies of people involved with AIDS and the practical aspects of medical, legal, and financial issues. Has an annotated bibliography and glossary.

Miller, David. **Living With AIDS and HIV.** Dobbs Ferry, NY: Macmillan Press/Sheridan House, 1987. 144 p. ISBN 0-333-43243-6; ISBN 0-333-43244-4 (pbk.).

Miller, David; Weber, Jonathan; and Green, John, eds. **The Management of AIDS Patients.** Basingstoke: Macmillan, 1986. 202p. ISBN 0-333-40465-3; ISBN 0-333-40466-1 (pbk.).

   A collection of articles covering the clinical and epidemiologal aspects of the disease.

National Academy of Sciences. Institute of Medicine. Committee on a National Strategy for AIDS. **Confronting AIDS: Directions for Public Health, Health Care and Research.** Washington DC: National Academy Press, 1986. 374p. ISBN 0-309-03699-2.

   An account of two public meetings and invited reports held by the Institute of Medicine of the National Academy of Sciences which provides an extensive overview of the complex aspects of AIDS.

National Academy of Sciences. Institute of Medicine. Eva K. Nichols, writer. **Mobilizing Against AIDS: The Unfinished Story of a Virus.** Cambridge, MA: Harvard University Press, 1986. 212 p. ISBN 0-674-57760-4; ISBN 0-674-57761-2 (pbk.).

   Summary of an annual meeting in October 1985 of the Institute of Medicine. Surveys knowledge of AIDS and issues raised by the disease.

Office of Technology Assessment. **Review of the Public Health Service's Response to AIDS.** Washington, DC: OTA, 1985. For sale by U.S. G.P.O. 158 p.

Pierce, Christine, and VanDeVeer, Donald, eds. **AIDS: Ethics and Public Policy.** Belmont, CA: Wadsworth Pub. Co., 1988. 241 p. ISBN 0-534-08286-6.

Population Reports - AIDS: A Public Health Crisis. Baltimore, MD: Population Information Program, The Johns Hopkins University, 1987.

Review many aspects of the AIDS situation including epidemiology. Can be ordered from the Population Information Program, The Johns Hopkins University, 624 N. Broadway, Baltimore, MD 21205.

Reports on AIDS Published in the Morbidity and Mortality Weekly Report: June 1981 Through February 1986. Atlanta, GA: Dept. of Health and Human Services, Public Health Service, Centers for Disease Control, 1986. 155 p.

Reprints from *MMWR.*

Selikoff, Irving J.; Teirstein, Alvin S.; and Hirschman, Shalom Z., eds. **Acquired Immune Deficiency Syndrome.** New York: New York Acacemy of Sciences, 1984. 622 p. ISBN 0-89766-268-7; ISBN 0-89766-269-5 (pbk.). (*Annals of the New York Acacemy of Sciences*, vol. 437.)

Staquet, M.; Hemmer, R.; and Baert, A., eds. **Clinical Aspects of AIDS and AIDS Related Complex.** Oxford; New York: Oxford University Press, 1986. 209 p. ISBN 0-19-261615-3.

A collection of articles that discuss international research studies.

Sunderland, Ronald, and Shelp, Earl E. **AIDS: A Manual for Pastoral Care.** Philadelphia: Westminster Press, 1987. ISBN 0-664-24088-7 (pbk.)

United States Conference of Mayors. **National Directory of AIDS-Related Services.** Washington, DC: The Conference, February 1986.

U.S. Department of Health and Human Services. Public Health Service. **AIDS Information/Education Plan to Prevent and Control AIDS in the U.S.** Bethesda, MD: U.S. Department of Health and Human Services, 1987.

Warshaw, Leon J., ed. **AIDS and The Employer: Guidelines on the Management of AIDS in the Workplace.** New York: New York Business Group on Health, Inc., 1986. 86 p.

Contains information concerning employers, legal considerations, costs of care, and medical problems.

Witt, Michael D., ed. **AIDS and Patient Management: Legal, Ethical and Social Issues.** Owings Mills, MD: National Health Publishing, 1986. 263p. ISBN 0-932500-46-3.

A collection of articles dealing with the legal, ethical and social issues of AIDS. Includes guidelines for the management of AIDS patients, much reprinted from *MMWR.*

Wormser, Gary P.; Stahl, Rosalyn; and Bottone, Edward J., eds. **AIDS-Acquired Immune Deficiency Syndrome-and Other Manifestations of HIV Infection.** Park Ridge, NJ: Noyes Publications, 1987. 1103 p. ISBN 0-8155-1108-6.

Written by over 100 contributors, this extensive volume contains over 3,000 references and authoritatively discusses numerous aspects of the disease.

Audiovisual Producers

Numerous audiovisual programs are being produced on the subject of AIDS with the most prevalent format being the videotape cassette. Titles in this listing are assumed to be available as videotapes unless otherwise noted. Programs have been listed according to the name of the producing organization so that the prospective user can contact that agency for the most up-to-date information on the cost of the audiovisual, availability, format, revised editions, and new products. Several resources for locating new material as it is developed include a free catalog from the National Audiovisual Center (see listing in this chapter) and the online database AVLINE, produced by the National Library of Medicine (see the chapter, Computerized Sources of Information).

ALL Media Productions
2839 Breton Road SE
Grand Rapids, MI 49506
(616) 459-9703

AIDS: Learn For Your Life 25 min

American College Health Association
15879 Crabbs Branch Way
Rockville, MD 20855
(301) 963-1100

The AIDS Dilemma: Higher Education's Response 90 min

American Journal of Nursing Company
Educational Services Division
555 West 57th Street
New York, NY 10019

(212) 582-8820
(212) 223-2282

> *AIDS: A Nursing Perspective*   29 min

American Public Health Association
1015 15th Street NW
Washington, DC 20005
(202) 789-5600

> *AIDS: Virology and Serology*
> *AIDS Education: Two Program Examples*
> *The Epidemic That Will Not Go Away: Public Health Policy Issues and
>   AIDS*
> *Public Health Promotion Policy: Description and Issues*
> *Women and AIDS*

American Red Cross
1730 D Street NW
Washington, DC 20006
(202) 737-8300

> *AIDS -- Spread Facts, Not Fear*   20 min   (slide/tape)
> *Beyond Fear*
>   *Part I. The Virus*   20 min
>   *Part II. The Individual*   20 min
>   *Part III. The Community*   20 min
> *A Letter From Brian*   28 min

Audio-Video Digest Foundation
1577 East Chevy Chase Drive
Glendale, CA 91206

> *The Epidemiology of Acquired Immune Deficiency Syndrome*   39 min
> *Immunology of Acquired Immune Deficiency Syndrome*   50 min
> *Kaposi's Sarcoma in Acquired Immune Deficiency Syndrome (AIDS)*
>   31 min
> *Treating the Gay Patient*   60 min

Boston Public Schools
Medical Services
26 Court Street
Boston, MA 02108
(617) 726-6200, ext. 5185

> *AIDS*   28 min

Career Aids
A Division of Opportunities for Learning, Inc.
20417 Nordhoff Street
Department 4
Chatsworth, CA 91311
(818) 341-8200

> *AIDS: Part I and Part II*   15 min each
> *AIDS: The Disease and What We Know*   20 min
> *AIDS: Our Worst Fears*   57 min
> *Stopping a Killer: The AIDS Antibody Test*   28 min

Carle Medical Communications
510 West Main Street
Urbana, IL 61801
(217) 384-4838

> *An Institutional Response to A.I.D.S.*   18 min (16mm also)
> *Overcoming Irrational Fear of AIDS*   22 min
> *Psychosocial Interventions in AIDS*   22 min

Carolina Biological Supply Company
2700 York Road
Burlington, NC 27215
(919) 584-0381
(800) 334-5551

> *AIDS*   20 min

Centers for Disease Control
1600 Clifton Road
Atlanta, GA 30307-0528

> *AIDS and Your Job: What Everyone Should Know About AIDS*   20
> min

Channing L. Bete Co., Inc.
200 State Road
South Deerfield, MA 01373
(413) 665-7611

Publishes multimedia on health-related topics including AIDS.

Churchill Films
662 North Robertson Boulevard
Los Angeles, CA 90069-9970
(800) 334-7830

> *AIDS -- What Everyone Needs To Know*   18 min
> *A Million Teenagers*   22 min

Cinema Group Home Video
1461 Amalfi Drive
Pacific Palisades, CA 90272

> *Safer Sex for Men & Women: How to Avoid Catching AIDS*   60 min

Communications Park
Box 1000
Mount Kisco, NY 10549-9989

> *AIDS: Facts and Fears, Crisis and Controversy*   23 min

Conus Communications
3415 University Avenue
Minneapolis, MN 55414
(612) 642-4645

> *The AIDS Connection*   5 hr. television presentation

Coronet Films and Video
108 Wilmot Road
Deerfield, IL 60015-9990
(312) 940-1260
(800) 621-2131

> *Nova: Can AIDS Be Stopped*   58 min
>   (transcript available from: Nova, Box 322, Boston, MA 02134 (800)
>   621-2131; Illinois or Alaska call collect (312) 940-1260)

Educational Productions
4925 S. W. Humphrey Park Crest
Portland, OR 97221
(503) 292-9234

The Legacy: A Series of Videos for Hospital Settings
    I. The Overview   30 min
    II. The Physician   30 min
    III. The Nurse   30 min
    IV. The Social Worker   30 min

Emory Medical Television Network
Emory University School of Medicine
Atlanta, GA 30322

Acquired Immune Deficiency Syndrome   48 min
AIDS, a Deck of Cards   58 min
AIDS, an Olde or New Acquaintance?   42 min
AIDS in the Pediatric Age Group   44 min
Clinical AIDS Conference   56 min
Clinical and Epidemiological Aspects of the HTLV-3 Infection   57 min
Nursing Care for Patients With AIDS   56 min
An Overview of AIDS and Human T-Cell Lymphocytotropic Virus-3 Infections   *41 min*
Serologic Testing HTLV-3 Infection: What the Clinician Should Know   44 min

Encyclopaedia Britannica
Education Corporation
425 North Michigan Avenue
Chicago, IL 60611

AIDS Alert   16 min

Fairview General Hospital
18101 Lorain Avenue
Cleveland, OH 44111
(216) 476-7000

AIDS Overview: Infection Control   14 min

Films for the Humanities and Sciences, Inc.
P. O. Box 2053
Princeton, NJ 08543
(800) 257-5126

AIDS: Are You at Risk?   19 min
AIDS: Our Worst Fears   57 min
AIDS and the Arts   20 min
AIDS Face to Face   28 min
Is Our Blood Supply Safe?   19 min

Not Ready to Die of AIDS 52 min
Safe Sex 28 min
Sexually-Transmitted Diseases 19 min
Women and AIDS 28 min

Films Incorporated
5547 North Ravenswood Avenue
Chicago, IL 60640-1199

In the Midst of Life 28 min
Life, Death, and AIDS 52 min
Main Street: Sex and American Teens 45 min
Men, Women, Sex and AIDS 49 min
Your Biological Guide to AIDS 25 min

Focus International
14 Oregon Drive
Huntington Station, NY 11746
(800) 843-0305
(516) 549-5320 (NY only)

AIDS Alert 23 min
For Our Lives 25 min

Gay Men's Health Crisis
Box 274, 132 West 24th Street
New York, NY 10011
(212) 807-7517

Chance of a Lifetime 43 min

Goodday Video Productions
115 North Esplanade Street
Cuero, TX 77954
800) 221-1426

AIDS: Suddenly Sex Has Become Very Dangerous
Part I. Overview 21 min
Part II. For Students 32 min
Part III. For Parents and Teachers 28 min

Health Education Services
10200 Jefferson Boulevard, Room H31
P. O. Box 802
Culver City, CA 90232-0802

Produces educational materials for grades 7 to 12, i.e. books, pamphlets, films, videos, wall charts, multimedia kits, etc. on health issues and problems including AIDS.

Hospital Satellite Network
San Francisco General Hospital Medical Center
1001 Potrero Avenue
San Francisco, CA 94110
(415) 821-8200

> *Caring for the AIDS Patient*   29 min
> *Management of the AIDS Patient*   60 min

Human Relations Media
175 Tompkins Avenue
Pleasantville, NY 10570
(800) 431-2050

> *AIDS: What Are the Risks?*   30 min (filmstrip/tape or filmstrip on video)

Indiana University Audiovisual Center
Bloomington, IN 47405
(812) 335-8087

> *AIDS: Profile of an Epidemic -- Update*   60 min

InfoMedix
12800 Garden Grove Boulevard
Suite F
Garden Grove, CA 92643

> Produces audiocassettes of the Third International Conference on AIDS held in Washington in June 1987.

KDFW-TV
400 North Griffin
Dallas, TX 75202
(214) 720-4444

> *AIDS Update*   55 min

Krames Communications
312 90th Street
Daly City, CA 94015-1898

Produces pamphlets, posters, microcomputer programs, and videotapes to promote employee and patient wellness, increase productivity, and reduce health care costs.

Marshfield Medical Foundation
St. Joseph's Hospital
611 St. Joseph Avenue
Marshfield, WI 54449
(715) 387-1713

AIDS 32 min
AIDS, the Widening Gyra 47 min
Opportunistic Infection in an Immune Compromise State 46 min

Medcom, Inc.
Public Health Laboratory
7077 Orangewood Avenue
Garden Grove, CA 92641

AIDS Program I -- Epidemiology 15 min (slide/tape)
AIDS Program II -- Infection Control 15 min (slide/tape)

Medical Action Group
P. O. Box 598
Chanute, KS 66720
(316) 431-0140
(800) 522-2437

The AIDS Video -- AIDS and the American Family 58 min

Modern Talking Picture Service
5000 Park Street North
St. Petersburg, FL 33709
(813) 541-5763

AIDS: Fears and Facts 24 min

MPI Home Video
15825 Rob Roy Drive

Oak Forest, IL 60452
(312) 687-7881

AIDS: Profile of an Epidemic -- Update 57 min

MTI Film and Video
108 Wilmot Road
Deerfield, IL 60015
(312) 940-1260
(800) 621-2131

AIDS: An ABC News Special 12 min
AIDS: Facts Over Fears 25 min
AIDS and the Health Care Worker 27 min

Multi-Focus
1525 Franklin Street
San Francisco, CA 94109
(415) 673-5100

AIDS and Health Education Series
  Approaching the Topic of AIDS 17 min
  Discussing Health Care and AIDS 17 min
  AIDS, Women and Sexuality 17 min
  AIDS, Men and Sexuality 17 min
  Living With AIDS Related Conditions 20 min
Norma and Tony: Following Safer Sex Guidelines 30 min

National Audiovisual Center
Information Services Park
8700 Edgeworth Drive
Capitol Heights, MD 20743-3701
(301) 763-1896
(800) 638-1300

Serves as the central distribution source for more than 8000 audiovisual programs produced by the U.S. government. A free catalog is available.

National Broadcasting Company, Inc.
Program Merchandising
1270 Avenue of Americas
New York, NY 10028
(212) 664-4444, ext.5031

An Early Frost　23 min
Life, Death, and AIDS　52 min

National Center for Homecare Education and Research
350 Fifth Avenue
New York, NY
(212) 560-3300

Living With AIDS　27 min

Network for Continuing Medical Education
15 Columbus Circle
New York, NY　10023
(212) 541-8088

Acquired Immune Deficiency Syndrome: AIDS　47 min
AIDS in the Hospital　30 min

New Day Films
22 Riverside Drive
Wayne, NJ　07470-3191
(201) 633-0212

The AIDS Movie　26 min　(16mm also)

New York Department of Health
Division of Health Promotion
125 Worth Street
Box 46
New York, NY　10013
(212) 566-7130

A Special Report on AIDS　90 min

ODN Productions, Inc.
74 Varick Street
Suite 304
New York, NY　10013
(212) 431-8923

Sex, Drugs, and AIDS　18 min
The Subject is AIDS　18 min

Perennial Education, Inc.
The Altschul Group
930 Pitner Avenue
Evanston, IL 60202

  AIDS in Your School   23 min

Pyramid Films
P. O. Box 1048
Santa Monica, CA 90406
(800) 421-2304
(213) 828-7577

  About AIDS   15 min   (16mm also)

San Francisco AIDS Foundation
25 Van Ness Street
San Francisco, CA 94102
(415) 864-4376
(415) 864-4376

  An Epidemic of Fear -- AIDS in the Workplace   23 min

Shanti Project
525 Howard Street
San Francisco, CA 94105
(415) 777-CARE

  AIDS Clients and Counselors Panel   57 min and 9 min
  AIDS Clinical Issues   48 min and 45 min
  AIDS Medical Overview   48 min
  AIDS Psychosocial Issues   58 min and 60 min
  Facilitating a Support Group   49 min
  Facing Death and Dying   26 min
  Fishbowl Roleplays   58 min
  Friends and Family Support Group   54 min
  Grieving Clients and Counselors Panel   57 min and 13 min
  How to Avoid Burnout   59 min
  Introduction to Grief   46 min
  Levels of Active Listening   60 min
  Patient Advocacy   35 min and 60 min
  People With AIDS Support Group   60 min and 24 min
  Shanti Counseling Approach   55 min
  Volunteer Counselors Support Groups   48 min

Time-Life Video
1271 Avenue of Americas
New York, NY 10020
(212) 484-5940

> *AIDS: Chapter One* 57 min

U.S. Public Health Service
Public Affairs Office
Hubert H. Humphrey Building
Room 725-H
200 Independence Avenue SW
Washington, DC 20201
(202) 245-6867

> *AIDS: Tracking the Mystery* 20 min
> *Facts About AIDS* (3 programs)
> *What If the Patient Has AIDS?* 20 min

Walt Disney Education Media Co.
500 South Buena Vista Street
Burbank, CA 91521
(800) 423-2555

> *A.I.D.S.* 18 min

WBZ-TV, Boston
c/o AIDS Action Committee
661 Boylston Street
Boston, MA 02116

> *AIDS Lifeline* 60 min

Workplace Health Communications Corporation
4 Madison Place
Albany,NY 12202
(518) 434-2381

> *Managing AIDS in the Workplace*

General Index

Geographic Index

NOTES

NOTES

NOTES